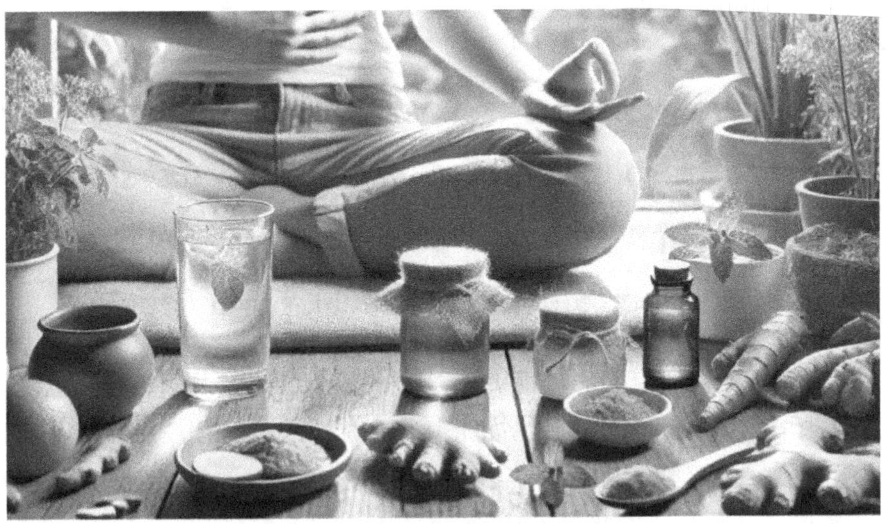

HEALING FROM
SIBO

A Step-by-Step Guide to Restoring Gut Health and Overcoming Small Intestinal Bacterial Overgrowth

Verna B. Hagen

COPYRIGHT PAGE

All rights reserved. No part of this publication may be reproduced, stored in a retrieval system, or transmitted in any form or by any means, whether electronic, mechanical, photocopying, recording, or otherwise, without the prior written consent of the publisher, except for brief excerpts used in reviews or scholarly commentary.

DISCLAIMER PAGE

This book is intended for educational purposes only and should not be considered a replacement for professional medical advice, diagnosis, or treatment. Before making any changes to your diet, exercise routine, or treatment plan, always consult with a healthcare professional.

The author and publisher are not liable for any negative outcomes or consequences arising from the use of the information in this book. Results may differ from person to person, and the content should not be used as a substitute for professional medical consultation.

SMALL INTESTINE BACTERIAL OVERGROWTH (SIBO)

Small intestine bacterial overgrowth (SIBO) is a condition in which there is an overgrowth of bacteria in the small intestine, leading to symptoms such as bloating, diarrhea, and malabsorption of nutrients.

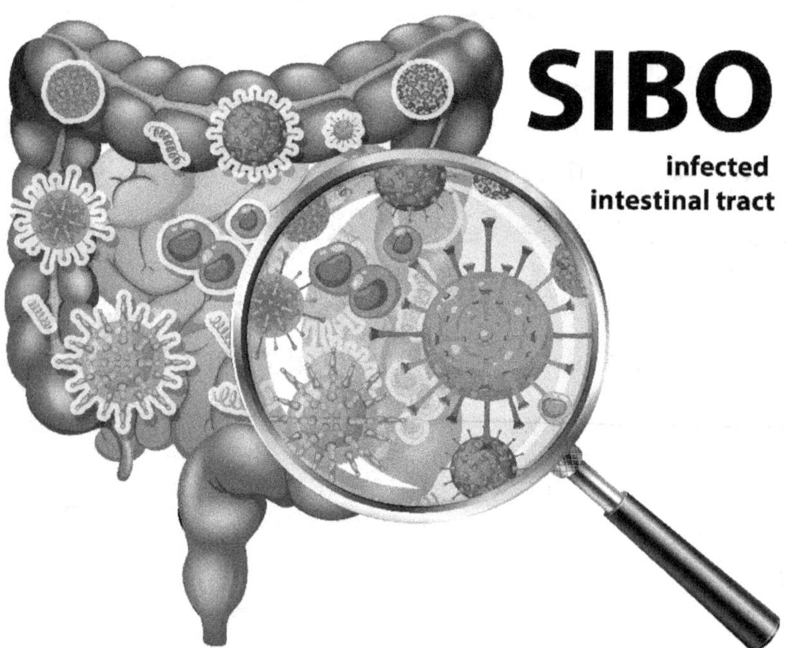

Table of Contents

Foreword

SIBO) is a condition that affects far more people than many realize. Its symptoms are often misunderstood, misdiagnosed, or dismissed as a part of everyday life. For anyone experiencing persistent digestive issues, fatigue, bloating, or brain fog, the path to understanding SIBO and how it impacts overall health can feel overwhelming.

In this book, I aim to provide you with an in-depth yet accessible guide to SIBO, from understanding the science behind the condition to practical, actionable steps for healing. Designed to help you reclaim control of your digestive health, offering not just knowledge, but a roadmap for recovery.

Through a combination of expert insights, personal success stories, and evidence-based strategies. The path to overcoming SIBO may be challenging, but with the right tools, mindset, and support, it's entirely within your reach.

Introduction

A Personal Journey with SIBO

Imagine this scenario: You've been struggling with bloating, cramps, and exhaustion for months. Despite seeing several doctors, trying various medications, and experimenting with different diets, nothing seems to work. Frustration builds, confusion sets in, and it starts to feel like you'll never return to a place of good health.

This was the experience of Sarah, a 32-year-old woman who came to me with severe digestive issues. After countless tests and visits to multiple specialists, Sarah was finally diagnosed with Small Intestinal Bacterial Overgrowth (SIBO), a condition where an excessive number of bacteria in the small intestine disrupts normal digestion. For years, Sarah had been enduring these debilitating symptoms—bloating, diarrhea, chronic fatigue, and mental fog—without knowing that they were all linked to this common yet often overlooked condition.

Just like Sarah, many people with SIBO struggle to understand what's causing their symptoms. Getting a clear diagnosis can be a lengthy and difficult process. Even once you have the diagnosis, the road to recovery can be filled with uncertainty.

The good news is that SIBO is manageable. By understanding its root causes and making strategic adjustments to your diet, lifestyle, and treatment plan, you can heal your gut, regain your vitality, and restore your health.

This book is here to guide you through that journey. With a clear, step-by-step method, I'll show you how to heal from SIBO, restore balance to your digestive system, and take back control of your health.

How to Use This Guide

This guide is designed to equip you with both the knowledge and practical tools necessary to conquer SIBO and restore your gut health. Whether you're new to a SIBO diagnosis or have been living with it for some time, this book will provide support and guidance throughout every stage of your healing process.

Start with the Basics

In the opening chapters, we'll break down what SIBO is, how it develops, and the common symptoms to look for. Understanding the underlying mechanisms is crucial for creating an effective recovery plan.

Diet and Nutrition

One of the key components of healing from SIBO is adjusting your diet. In Chapter 2, we'll take a deep dive into the foods that can either help or hinder your recovery, with an emphasis on popular dietary strategies like the Low FODMAP diet and Specific Carbohydrate Diet (SCD). You'll also find practical meal planning advice and easy-to-follow recipes to help restore balance to your digestive system.

The 25-Day Healing Plan

At the core of this book is the 25-Day Healing Plan, a step-by-step program designed to help you rebuild your gut health each day. This plan includes a balanced approach, integrating dietary changes, supplements, lifestyle shifts, and self-care practices, making it straightforward and actionable.

Lifestyle Tips for Long-Term Success

Healing from SIBO involves more than just diet—it's about creating sustainable habits that support ongoing gut health. In the later chapters, we'll explore essential lifestyle factors like managing stress, improving sleep, staying active, and other wellness practices that contribute to long-term digestive health.

This book is your guide, your blueprint, and your partner in navigating the path to better health. Healing from SIBO takes patience and consistency, but with the right approach, you can restore your gut health and regain your vitality.

Take it step by step, and remember that you don't
have to do this alone. By following the plan laid out
in this book, you'll be on the road to recovery.

Chapter 1

What is SIBO?

SIBO stands for "small intestinal bacterial overgrowth." This is a situation in which too many bacteria grow in the small intestine. There are usually a lot fewer bugs in the small intestine than in the large intestine. This is because the small intestine is mostly responsible for absorbing nutrients.

But in people with SIBO, bacteria from the large intestine move to the small intestine or grow in a way that isn't usual. This makes digestion and nutrient absorption more difficult.

Food ferments in the small intestine when there are too many bacteria. This makes gas and causes symptoms like pain, bloating, diarrhoea, and constipation. Also, these germs can make it harder for the body to absorb important nutrients like vitamin B12, iron, and fat-soluble vitamins, which can lead to nutritional deficiencies.

SIBO can have many different reasons, but some of them are:

- Gut motility problems (like those seen in people with IBS, diabetes, or history of surgery);
- Problems with the structure of the digestive tract (like diverticula or adhesions)
- Weakened immune system or imbalances in the gut bacteria
- Long-term use of antibiotics or other drugs that hurt gut health

Breath tests are usually used to make the diagnosis. These tests measure the gases that are made when bacteria ferment food.

SIBO can be treated with antibiotics, changes to the diet, and sometimes probiotics. But to keep it under control in the long run, you need to do more than that, like healing the gut lining and balancing the microbiome.

The Importance of Gut Health

Gut health is foundational to general health. Your gut system does more than just break down food. It also absorbs nutrients, keeps your immune system in check, and affects your mental and emotional health.

In fact, approximately 70% of your immune system is found in your gut, highlighting its role in protecting the body against harmful pathogens and diseases.

The gut also plays a vital role in producing neurotransmitters like serotonin, which is crucial for mood control. Studies show that a significant amount of serotonin (around 90%) is made in the gut, which is why digestive health is so closely linked to mental health.

A balanced gut microbiome (the community of bacteria and other microorganisms in your intestines) supports everything from digestion and immune function to cognitive health and mental stability.

When the balance of bacteria in the gut is disrupted—whether by SIBO, poor diet, or other factors—it can lead to a cascade of problems. These include digestive problems, nutritional deficiencies, inflammation, and even mental health concerns like anxiety and sadness. This is why restoring gut health is so crucial not only for healing from SIBO but for general well-being.

How SIBO Affects Your Body and Mind

SIBO doesn't just cause gut symptoms—it can affect the entire body and mind in complex ways. Because it disrupts nutrient absorption, it can lead to a variety of nutritional deficiencies, which in turn can affect energy levels, brain function, and general vitality. Here's how SIBO impacts both the body and the mind:

Physical Effects:

1. ***Bloating and Gas:*** When bacteria in the small intestine ferment food improperly, they make

gases like hydrogen and methane. These gases collect and cause uncomfortable bloating and distension in the abdomen.

2. ***Diarrhea or Constipation:*** The disrupted digestion and changed motility can cause either diarrhea (due to malabsorption of fats and bile acids) or constipation (due to slowed gut motility).

3. ***Nutrient Deficiencies:*** As the overgrowth of bacteria stops proper digestion, key nutrients like vitamin B12, iron, calcium, and magnesium may not be absorbed effectively, leading to deficiencies.

4. ***Fatigue:*** Nutrient malabsorption, mixed with the chronic inflammation that SIBO can cause, can leave you feeling constantly tired and sluggish.

Mental and Emotional Impact:

1. ***Brain Fog:*** One of the most frustrating symptoms of SIBO is brain fog, a cognitive impairment that makes it hard to focus or think clearly. This can be linked to both the nutritional deficiencies caused by SIBO and the inflammatory processes happening in the gut.

2. ***Mood Swings and Anxiety***: The gut-brain link is a well-established pathway. An imbalanced gut microbiome can add to symptoms of anxiety, depression, and mood swings. The presence of harmful bacteria in the small intestine may cause inflammation, which can negatively affect the brain and alter mood-regulating chemicals like serotonin.

3. ***Depression:*** People with chronic digestive problems like SIBO may also experience depression as a result of prolonged discomfort, disrupted daily life, and a sense of isolation.

There's growing evidence that a compromised gut microbiome can add to depressive symptoms.

SIBO's effects reach far beyond the digestive system. For many people, the mental and emotional toll of living with chronic symptoms can be just as challenging as the physical discomfort. Understanding this connection is key to fully addressing the effect of SIBO and restoring health to both body and mind.

Chapter 2

Understanding SIBO

The Science Behind SIBO

Small Intestinal Bacterial Overgrowth (SIBO) is a disease where there is an abnormal increase in the number of bacteria in the small intestine. Normally, the small intestine has only a small number of bacteria, as most of the digestive system's bacteria live in the large intestine. However, in people with SIBO, these bacteria overpopulate the small intestine and begin to interfere with digestion and nutrient absorption.

The excess bacteria can also ferment undigested food, creating gas and leading to uncomfortable symptoms like bloating and cramping.

The small intestine's main job is to break down food and absorb nutrients, and when bacteria disrupt this process, the balance of the gut microbiome is altered, leading to digestive distress.

Understanding the underlying science is important for creating an effective treatment plan.

Types of SIBO: Hydrogen, Methane, and Mixed SIBO

There are three main types of SIBO, classified by the type of gases released by the overgrown bacteria: Hydrogen SIBO, Methane SIBO, and Mixed SIBO.

1. Hydrogen SIBO: This is the most common type of SIBO. The overgrowth of bacteria in the small intestine creates hydrogen gas as a byproduct of fermentation. This can lead to signs such as bloating, diarrhea, and cramping.

2. Methane SIBO: In this type, methane gas is made by the bacteria in the small intestine. Methane SIBO is often linked with constipation and other more severe digestive symptoms. It can also affect the motility of the intestines, causing slow digestion and further pain.

3. Mixed SIBO: As the name suggests, this type includes the production of both hydrogen and methane gases. The symptoms are a combination of those seen in hydrogen and methane SIBO and can vary in intensity.

Understanding the specific type of SIBO you have is crucial for determining the most effective treatment approach, as each type may react differently to dietary changes, antibiotics, and other interventions.

Symptoms of SIBO

The symptoms of SIBO can vary from person to person, but they typically include:

1. ***Bloating:*** One of the hallmark signs of SIBO, caused by the fermentation of leftover food by bacteria.

2. ***Abdominal Pain and Cramping:*** Often a result of the bacteria making gas and fermenting food in the small intestine.

3. ***Diarrhea or Constipation:*** Depending on the type of SIBO, you may experience either

frequent, watery stools (hydrogen SIBO) or slow digestion leading to constipation (methane SIBO).

4. ***Fatigue:*** As the gut becomes unbalanced, your body may not receive nutrients properly, leading to feelings of exhaustion.

5. ***Brain Fog:*** The gut-brain link can make you feel mentally foggy or less focused. Because these symptoms overlap with many other digestive diseases, diagnosing SIBO requires specific tests and procedures, which we'll cover later in the chapter.

Causes of SIBO: Diet, Lifestyle, and Medical Factors

Several factors can add to the development of SIBO, ranging from dietary habits to medical conditions:

1. ***Dietary Factors:*** A diet high in sugar and processed foods can cause bacterial overgrowth. Additionally, certain food intolerances, such as lactose or fructose, may worsen symptoms.

2. ***Lifestyle Factors:*** Chronic stress, inadequate sleep, and lack of physical exercise can disrupt the normal motility of the digestive system, creating an environment conducive to bacterial overgrowth.

3. ***Medical Factors:*** Certain conditions like irritable bowel syndrome (IBS), celiac disease, Crohn's disease, and previous gastrointestinal surgeries can increase the risk of getting SIBO. A disease known as motility disorder, where the small intestine fails to move food properly, is also a common underlying cause.

A combination of these factors often leads to the growth of SIBO, and addressing them is key to healing.

How to Diagnose SIBO: Tests and Procedures

The most reliable way to identify SIBO is through breath tests, which measure the gases produced by bacteria in the small intestine.

1. ***Lactulose Breath Test:*** This test involves swallowing a sugar called lactulose, which is not absorbed by the body. If bacteria in the small intestine ferment it, they make hydrogen or methane gases, which are then measured in your breath. Elevated levels of these gases suggest SIBO.

2. ***Glucose Breath Test:*** Similar to the lactulose test, the glucose test uses a sugar solution to

measure hydrogen or methane levels. This test can be more accurate for diagnosing SIBO because glucose is absorbed more quickly, giving a better indication of bacterial overgrowth in the small intestine.

In some cases, additional testing, such as stool analysis or endoscopy, may be suggested, but breath tests remain the gold standard for diagnosing SIBO.

Chapter 3

The Importance of Diet in SIBO Recovery

The Role of Diet in Gut Health

Diet plays a key role in managing and recovering from Small Intestinal Bacterial Overgrowth (SIBO). Your gut is a complex ecosystem of bacteria, viruses, fungi, and other microbes, all of which impact your digestion, immune system, and general health. In a healthy gut, beneficial bacteria work in harmony to break down food and collect nutrients. However, when there is an overgrowth of harmful bacteria in the small intestine, it disrupts this process, leading to digestive discomfort, malabsorption of nutrients, and inflammation.

Diet can either add to or alleviate this imbalance. For people with SIBO, the foods you eat can have a profound effect on the bacterial balance in your gut. Some foods fuel the overgrowth of harmful bacteria, worsening symptoms, while others can help restore balance by boosting gut healing, reducing inflammation, and supporting digestion.

The key is to understand which foods are helpful and which ones exacerbate the condition. By following a targeted dietary plan, you can reduce symptoms like bloating, abdominal pain, fatigue, and brain fog, and help create an environment in your gut that supports healing.

Foods to Avoid: What Makes SIBO Worse

When you have SIBO, your small intestine becomes overwhelmed with bacteria that ferment food, making gas and causing discomfort. Certain foods provide the perfect fuel for this bacterial fermentation, worsening symptoms and lengthening the condition. Avoiding these foods is important for reducing bacterial overgrowth and promoting healing.

1. High-FODMAP Foods

FODMAP means for Fermentable Oligosaccharides, Disaccharides, Monosaccharides, and Polyols, a group of short-chain carbohydrates that are poorly absorbed in the small intestine. These include many fruits, vegetables, dairy goods, and grains. When these foods are eaten, they ferment in the small intestine, feeding harmful bacteria and causing bloating, gas, and cramping.

Examples of high-FODMAP foods to avoid:

- ***Fruits:*** Apples, pears, watermelon, cherries, and stone fruits like peaches and plums
- ***Vegetables:*** Onions, garlic, cauliflower, broccoli, artichokes, and asparagus
- ***Dairy:*** Milk, soft cheeses, and yogurt (due to lactose)
- ***Grains and Legumes:*** Wheat, rye, chickpeas, lentils, and kidney beans
- ***Sweeteners:*** Sorbitol, mannitol, and high-fructose corn syrup

2. Processed and Refined Foods

Processed foods, which often contain added sugars, preservatives, and artificial sweeteners, can exacerbate SIBO symptoms by disrupting the gut microbiome and adding to inflammation. These foods may also be difficult to digest, putting additional strain on the already compromised digestive system.

Examples include

Fast food, sugary snacks, pre-packaged meals, and processed foods.

3. Gluten and Dairy (For Some Individuals)

While not everyone with SIBO is sensitive to gluten or dairy, many people with this condition find that cutting out these foods can help reduce symptoms. Gluten is found in wheat, barley, and rye, and can add to inflammation, while dairy can exacerbate symptoms if you have lactose intolerance, which is common in people with SIBO.

4. Alcohol and Caffeine

Alcohol, especially in excess, can irritate the gut lining and disrupt gut motility, possibly worsening SIBO symptoms. Caffeine, especially in large amounts, can also irritate the digestive system and lead to symptoms like diarrhea or abdominal cramping.

5. Legumes and Certain Vegetables

While vegetables are generally good for gut health, some vegetables, such as those high in fermentable fiber (e.g., beans, peas, and lentils), can worsen bloating and discomfort for individuals with SIBO. High-fiber veggies like onions, garlic, and cruciferous vegetables can be problematic as well.

Foods to Embrace: What Helps Heal SIBO

While avoiding certain foods is important in managing SIBO, there are many healing foods you can add into your diet that can help restore balance to your gut and alleviate symptoms. These foods are easy to process, low in fermentable carbohydrates, and support the growth of beneficial bacteria in the gut.

1. Lean Proteins

Lean meats like chicken, turkey, and fish are excellent sources of protein that are easy to digest and unlikely to drive bacterial overgrowth. They help repair the gut lining and provide important nutrients without causing irritation.

2. Non-Starchy Vegetables

Vegetables like spinach, zucchini, kale, carrots, and bell peppers are low in FODMAPs and provide important vitamins and minerals without feeding harmful bacteria. They are easy to digest and help support gut health.

3. Healthy Fats

Healthy fats from sources like olive oil, avocado, and coconut oil can help reduce inflammation in the gut and support the absorption of fat-soluble vitamins like A, D, E, and K. Fats also provide an energy source without overburdening the digestive system.

4. Bone Broth

Bone broth is rich in collagen and amino acids, which help repair the gut lining and lower inflammation. It is soothing for the digestive system and helps overall gut healing. It is also an excellent source of minerals like calcium, magnesium, and iron.

5. Fermented Foods (Carefully)

Fermented foods like kimchi, sauerkraut, and kefir contain helpful probiotics that can help restore a healthy balance of gut bacteria. However, it's important to add fermented foods slowly, as they can sometimes cause bloating and discomfort in the early stages of SIBO recovery. Start with small amounts and watch how your body responds.

6. Gluten-Free Grains (For Some)

Grains like rice, quinoa, and oats can be good options for individuals with SIBO, as they are usually well tolerated and low in FODMAPs. They provide essential fiber and nutrients without adding to fermentation in the small intestine.

7. Herbal Teas

Certain herbal teas, such as peppermint, ginger, and chamomile, have soothing effects on the digestive system and can help ease symptoms like bloating, nausea, and cramping. These teas can support digestion and improve gut motility.

The Low-FODMAP Diet: What You Need to Know

The Low-FODMAP diet is one of the most researched and successful dietary strategies for managing SIBO. As stated earlier, FODMAPs are a group of carbohydrates that are poorly absorbed in the small intestine. By reducing high-FODMAP foods, the diet aims to limit bacterial fermentation and reduce symptoms of bloating, gas, and cramping.

How the Low-FODMAP Diet Works

The Low-FODMAP diet is organized in three phases:

1. *Elimination Phase:* During this phase, you remove all high-FODMAP foods for about 4 to 6 weeks. This gives your gut time to heal and reduces the food source for the bacteria.

2. *Reintroduction Phase:* Once your symptoms have better, you begin reintroducing high-FODMAP foods one at a time. This allows you to identify which specific foods cause your symptoms.

3. *Personalization Phase:* After the reintroduction phase, you create a long-term eating plan that includes only those high-FODMAP foods that you accept, while avoiding the ones that cause symptoms.

Benefits of the Low-FODMAP Diet

The Low-FODMAP diet has been shown to greatly reduce symptoms of bloating, gas, diarrhea, and abdominal pain in many individuals with SIBO. It is often called the gold standard for SIBO management and is widely used by dietitians and healthcare professionals.

The Specific Carbohydrate Diet (SCD) vs. Low FODMAP: Pros and Cons

Both the Specific Carbohydrate Diet (SCD) and the Low-FODMAP diet are good dietary approaches for managing SIBO. However, they vary in their approach to food restrictions and the types of foods that are emphasized.

The Specific Carbohydrate Diet (SCD): The SCD removes all complex carbohydrates, including grains, starchy vegetables, and lactose. It focuses on simple carbohydrates that are easily absorbed by the body, like fruits, non-starchy veggies, and meat. The SCD is often used for diseases like Crohn's disease, IBS, and SIBO.

Pros of the SCD:

- Can help lower inflammation and support gut healing.
- Focuses on whole, raw foods.
- Effective for those with food allergies to grains and lactose.

Cons of the SCD:

- Very restrictive, especially for people who are used to a variety diet.
- Can be tough to follow long-term.

- Requires careful meal planning to ensure healthy balance.

The Low-FODMAP Diet:

As explained earlier, the Low-FODMAP diet focuses on reducing fermentable carbohydrates to minimize bacterial overgrowth. It is less restrictive than the SCD but still eliminates a large number of foods during the elimination phase.

Pros of the Low-FODMAP Diet:

- Has strong scientific proof supporting its effectiveness for SIBO.
- Easier to follow for those who need to keep a more varied diet.
- Can be customized based on individual triggers.

Cons of the Low-FODMAP Diet:

- The elimination phase can be difficult, as many common foods are restricted.
- Requires close attention to portion sizes and food combinations.

Diet is a cornerstone of managing **SIBO** and can play a major role in recovery. By avoiding foods that fuel bacterial overgrowth and incorporating foods that support gut healing, you can greatly reduce symptoms and improve your quality of life. Whether you choose the Low-FODMAP plan, the Specific Carbohydrate plan, or another dietary strategy, it is important to tailor your approach to your individual needs.

Always work with a healthcare provider, especially a registered dietitian, to ensure that your food supports your long-term health goals.

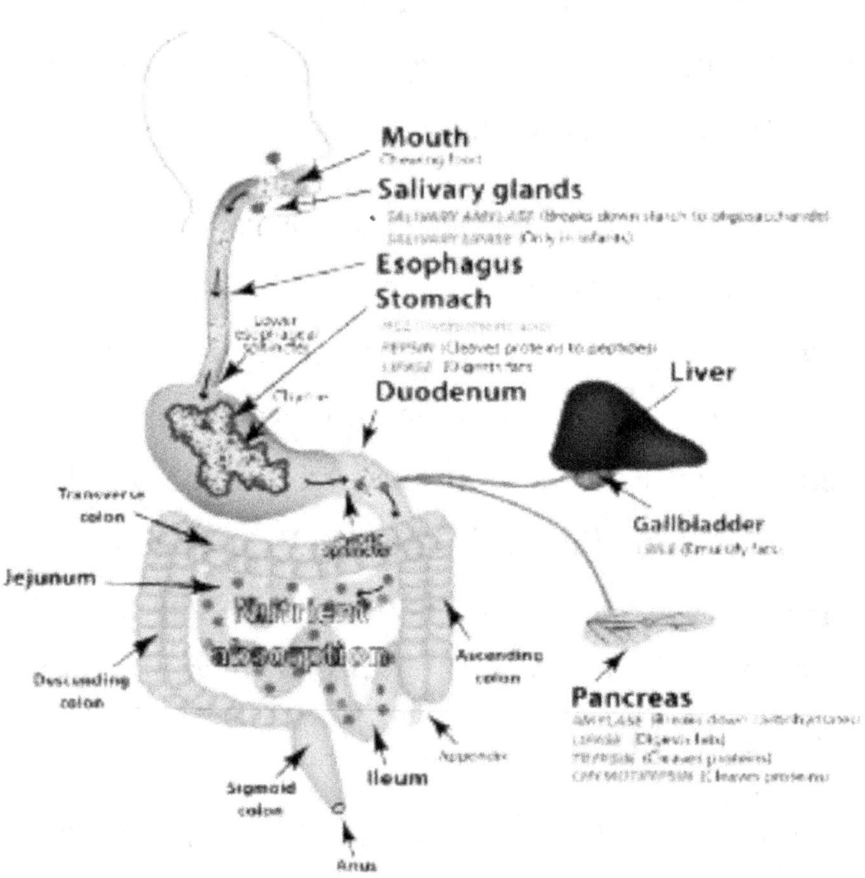

Mouth
Salivary glands
Esophagus
Stomach
Duodenum
Liver
Gallbladder
Transverse colon
Jejunum
Descending colon
Sigmoid colon
Anus
Ileum
Appendix
Ascending colon
Pancreas

Chapter 4

The 25-Day Healing Plan

The first five days of your SIBO healing journey are important. These days are about setting the foundation for your recovery by preparing your gut, detoxifying your body, and gently cleansing your digestive system. It's important to start slow and steady, allowing your body to adjust to new dietary patterns, supplements, and lifestyle changes. This phase sets the tone for the next stages of healing.

Day 1-5: Foundation Phase – Preparing for SIBO Recovery

The Foundation Phase (Days 1-5) is a preparatory period where your body begins to recalibrate and your gut starts the process of recovery. This phase focuses on lowering inflammation, improving digestion, and eliminating foods that may be exacerbating the overgrowth of bacteria. Think of these first five days as the "reset" phase—a time to cleanse your system and create healthy habits that will pave the way for a more complete healing process.

During these first few days, your main goals are to:

- Reduce bacterial load in the gut.
- Calm inflammation and irritation in the digestive tract.
- Begin balancing your gut microbiome with the right foods and supplements.

- Improve your body's ability to digest and receive nutrients.

Note: Healing from SIBO is a process that needs time and patience. It's important not to rush through these initial days, as setting a solid foundation is key to the success of the following phases.

Detoxing and Preparing Your Gut

Before you start actively targeting SIBO with treatments like antibiotics, herbs, or other therapies, it's important to detoxify your body gently and prepare your gut for healing. A detox doesn't mean extreme cleanses or fasting. Instead, it's about easing your digestive system into a healthier state by eliminating toxins and lowering inflammation.

Key Steps to Detoxing Your Gut:

1. Increase Hydration

Hydration is important to gut health. Water helps flush out toxins, support digestion, and keeps your gut lining hydrated. Aim for at least 8 cups of water a day, adding a pinch of Himalayan salt to support electrolyte balance. Warm water with a squeeze of lemon is a great choice to stimulate digestion in the morning.

2. Eliminate Processed Foods

Over the next five days, remove any processed foods, refined sugars, and artificial additives from your diet. These foods are inflammatory and can trigger gut dysbiosis (microbial imbalance), which is a key factor in SIBO. Instead, focus on nutrient-dense, whole foods like veggies, lean proteins, and healthy fats.

3. Start with Gut-Healing Foods

Incorporate foods that support the repair of the gut lining, such as bone broth, which is rich in collagen and amino acids that soothe and heal the digestive system. Cooked non-starchy vegetables like zucchini, spinach, and carrots are easy to digest and provide important vitamins and minerals.

4. Eliminate Dairy (If Applicable)

If you're sensitive to dairy or lactose, this is a good time to eliminate it from your diet to avoid further irritation to your gut lining. Dairy can contribute to bloating, inflammation, and exacerbate SIBO symptoms in some people.

How to Cleanse Your Body Without Drastic Measures

Cleansing your body doesn't take extreme measures or fasting. Instead, a gentle, balanced approach will allow your digestive system to reset without causing additional stress on your body. Here's how to cleanse effectively:

1. Focus on Whole Foods

Stick to nutrient-dense foods that support your liver and digestive organs in detoxification, such as leafy greens, beets, artichokes, and cruciferous veggies. These foods provide antioxidants and fiber that support natural detoxification processes.

2. Increase Fiber Intake

While fiber can sometimes cause bloating in the early stages of healing, soluble fiber is gentle on the digestive system and helps to keep things moving. Good sources include oats, chia seeds, and raw apples. However, you should avoid insoluble fiber at this time, as it may irritate the gut.

3. Incorporate Gentle Herbal Teas

Herbal teas such as peppermint, ginger, and chamomile are excellent for soothing the digestive system and stimulating digestive enzymes. They can help reduce bloating, ease pain, and promote better digestion, especially after meals.

4. Mindful Eating

During these days, take time to focus on your eating habits. Eat slowly, chew your food fully, and avoid distractions like screens. This mindful approach can help your body process food more efficiently, reducing the burden on your digestive system.

Daily Meal Plans (Low FODMAP / SCD)

During the Foundation Phase, it's important to stick to an anti-inflammatory diet, focusing on foods that promote healing while eliminating those that may cause irritation or worsen SIBO symptoms. Both the Low FODMAP Diet and the Specific Carbohydrate Diet (SCD) are effective approaches. Here's a breakdown of what to eat for the next five days:

Sample Daily Meal Plan (Day 1-5):

Day 1:

• **Breakfast:**

  o Scrambled eggs with spinach and a side of steamed zucchini

• **Lunch:**

- o Grilled chicken breast with a side of roasted carrots and quinoa (small amount)
- **Dinner:**
  - o Baked salmon with sautéed kale and olive oil
  - o Snack: A handful of pumpkin seeds or a boiled egg

Day 2: •

- **Breakfast:**
  - o Smoothie with almond milk, chia seeds, a small amount of strawberries, and a scoop of collagen powder
- **Lunch:**
  - o Turkey lettuce wraps with avocado, cucumber, and olive oil dressing
- **Dinner:**

o   Grass-fed beef stir-fry with bell peppers, spinach, and coconut oil

o   Snack: A small dish of cooked carrots or cucumber slices with a little hummus (low FODMAP)

Day 3:

- **Breakfast:**
  - o   Coconut yogurt (unsweetened) with chia seeds and blueberries
- **Lunch:**
  - o Grilled shrimp with sautéed zucchini andolive oil
- **Dinner:**
  - o   Bone broth soup with well-cooked non-starchy greens like spinach and carrots
  - o   Snack: Hard-boiled egg or a handful of walnuts

Day 4:

- **Breakfast:**
    - o Omelette with spinach, bell peppers, and olive oil
- **Lunch:**
    - o Grilled chicken with roasted sweet potatoes (small amount) and steamed asparagus
- **Dinner:**
    - o Baked cod with a side of roasted squash and arugula salad
    - o Snack: Carrot sticks with homemade guacamole

Day 5:

- **Breakfast:**
    - o Smoothie with kale, avocado, a few berries, and coconut milk

- **Lunch:**
  - Grass-fed beef with sautéed mushrooms (small amount) and green beans
- **Dinner:**
  - Grilled turkey with zucchini and mashed cauliflower (no dairy)
  - Snack: A handful of sunflower seeds or an apple (peeled)

Supplements to Support Your Gut Health

During the Foundation Phase, supplements can play a helpful role in the healing process. Supplements should be tailored to your individual needs and should not replace a healthy diet, but they can help reduce symptoms, support detoxification, and promote gut healing.

Here are some supplements that may be helpful during these first few days:

1. *Probiotics*

Probiotics help support the growth of beneficial bacteria in the gut, which is important for individuals with SIBO. Choose a high-quality, multi-strain probiotic that includes species like Lactobacillus and Bifidobacterium. However, be careful, as some people with SIBO experience increased bloating when taking probiotics in the early stages. Start with small amounts.

2. *Digestive Enzymes*

Digestive enzymes can help break down food more quickly, taking the burden off your digestive system. Look for a product that includes enzymes such as amylase, protease, and lipase, which help digest carbs, proteins, and fats respectively.

3. L-Glutamine

 L-glutamine is an amino acid that helps heal the gut lining, lower inflammation, and improve gut permeability. It's especially helpful for those with intestine permeability (leaky gut) or inflammation caused by SIBO.

4. Herbal Antimicrobials (If Recommended by Your Healthcare Provider)

Herbal antimicrobial supplements such as oregano oil, berberine, or allicin (garlic extract) can help lower bacterial overgrowth in the small intestine. It's important to work with a healthcare provider before incorporating these into your plan, as they can be potent and need to be used at the right time.

5. Magnesium

Magnesium supports muscle function, helps prevent constipation, and has a calming effect on the body. If you're having constipation (common in SIBO), magnesium citrate or magnesium glycinate can be helpful.

SIBO recovery plan are about building a solid foundation for your healing. By detoxing gently, setting up a diet plan tailored to your needs, and using the right supplements, you'll be preparing your body for greater healing. It's important to take it slow and listen to your body. Each day, make small but steady progress toward restoring balance to your gut. By the end of this phase, you'll have set the stage for the next steps in your journey to healing.

Day 6-10: Stabilization Phase – Strengthening Your Gut

The Stabilization Phase focuses on healing and strengthening your gut lining, managing any residual symptoms, establishing key lifestyle changes to support gut health. Each day has a specific focus, and the goal is to build upon the foundation you created in the first five days.

Day 6: Healing Your Gut Lining – Starting Strong

Focus: Healing the gut lining with anti-inflammatory foods and supplements.

Daily Tasks:

- **Morning:**

- o Drink a glass of water with the juice of half a lemon (supports liver detox).

  - o Take **L-Glutamine** (5 grams) to support gut lining repair.

  - o Eat a breakfast rich in **healthy fats** and **protein** (e.g., avocado and scrambled eggs with spinach).

- **Meals:**

  - o **Lunch:** Grilled chicken or turkey with steamed broccoli and cauliflower (both are anti-inflammatory and healing for the gut lining).

  - o **Snack:** Bone broth (1-2 cups) to provide collagen and amino acids that promote gut healing.

- **Evening:**

- Relax with a cup of **ginger tea** or **peppermint tea** to soothe any remaining digestive discomfort.

- Take a **digestive enzyme** supplement with dinner.

Supplementation: L-Glutamine, digestive enzymes, and collagen-rich bone broth.

Day 7: Managing Symptoms – Reducing Bloating and Gas

Focus: Addressing bloating, gas, and any digestive discomfort by continuing with dietary restrictions and supplement support.

Daily Tasks:

- **Morning:**

- o Start your day with **warm water** and a tablespoon of **apple cider vinegar** (diluted in water) to stimulate digestion.

- o Take **probiotic supplements** (if prescribed by your healthcare provider), to support gut flora balance.

- **Meals:**

  - o **Lunch:** A mixed greens salad with cucumber, avocado, grilled salmon, and olive oil dressing. This provides anti-inflammatory properties, omega-3 fatty acids, and fiber for digestive health.

  - o **Dinner:** A bowl of **bone broth** with sautéed kale and mushrooms.

- **Evening:**

  - Sip on **chamomile tea** or **fennel tea** to calm the digestive system before bed.

Supplementation: Probiotics (if applicable), digestive enzymes.

Day 8: Incorporating Detoxifying Foods – Cleansing and Restoring Balance

Focus: Adding detoxifying foods to support the liver, digestive tract, and overall recovery.

Daily Tasks:

- **Morning:**

  - Start with a **green smoothie** containing kale, cucumber, lemon juice, and ginger (excellent for detoxification).

- o Take your **L-Glutamine** to support gut health.

- **Meals:**

  - o **Lunch: Baked salmon** with steamed asparagus and quinoa (asparagus is a prebiotic and supports gut health).

  - o **Snack: Cucumber slices** with a tablespoon of olive oil and a sprinkle of sea salt (hydrating and detoxifying).

- **Evening:**

  - o Before bed, have a **gentle herbal tea** like peppermint or ginger to aid digestion.

Supplementation: L-Glutamine, digestive enzymes, and probiotics (if prescribed).

Day 9: Reducing Inflammation – Focus on Anti-Inflammatory Foods

Focus: Further reducing inflammation through diet and lifestyle practices.

Daily Tasks:

- **Morning:**

    o Drink a cup of **warm water with lemon** and a tablespoon of **apple cider vinegar** to start your digestion off right.

    o Add **turmeric powder** to your morning smoothie or drink a cup of **turmeric tea** (anti-inflammatory properties).

- **Meals:**

  - Lunch: A small serving of **grass-fed beef** or **lamb** with roasted zucchini, sweet potatoes, and spinach (rich in omega-3 and antioxidants).

  - Dinner: A bowl of **bone broth** with kale and a small portion of quinoa or rice for additional fiber.

- **Evening:**

  - Try a **relaxing yoga routine** or some light stretching before bed to reduce stress and promote digestion.

Supplementation: L-Glutamine, omega-3 supplements, turmeric.

Day 10: Optimizing Gut Function – Stress Reduction and Sleep

Focus: Supporting gut function with stress management and sleep optimization, while continuing dietary support.

Daily Tasks:

- **Morning:**

  - Start your day with **a cup of warm lemon water** and **apple cider vinegar**.

  - Take your **L-Glutamine** and **digestive enzyme** supplements.

- **Meals:**

  - **Lunch:** A bowl of **chicken soup** (bone broth-based) with leafy greens and herbs like parsley and thyme.

- o **Snack: Avocado** slices with a drizzle of olive oil (healthy fats support gut health).

- **Evening:**

  - o Wind down with **relaxation techniques** such as **deep breathing** or **meditation** to prepare for restful sleep.

  - o Enjoy a **herbal tea** (chamomile or peppermint) to help your digestive system relax before bed.

Supplementation: L-Glutamine, digestive enzymes, and omega-3 fatty acids.

Key Points for Days 6-10:

- **Gut Healing:** Continue with gut-healing foods and supplements (bone broth, L-Glutamine, probiotics, etc.).

- **Symptom Management:** Address residual symptoms (bloating, gas) with appropriate foods, teas, and supplements.

- **Lifestyle Focus:** Emphasize stress management, sleep, and light exercise to support overall healing.

- **Detoxification:** Incorporate detoxifying foods (like cruciferous vegetables, beets, and lemon) to support liver function and digestive health.

By Day 10, you should be noticing significant improvements in your gut function. While you may still experience some symptoms, the foundation you've laid during this Stabilization Phase will prepare you for more intensive healing in the next phases of your recovery plan.

Day 11-15: Restoration Phase – Rebuilding Gut Flora

One of the most important stages of your **recovery process** is the **Restoration Phase**. Your digestive system should be more stable by now, and the first phases of healing have laid the groundwork for your gut microbiota to return to equilibrium. The emphasis during this phase changes to the gradual reintroduction of foods, the use of probiotics and prebiotics to support gut flora, and the continuation of lifestyle choices that support gut health over the long term.

Day 11: How to Reintroduce Foods Slowly

Focus: Gradually reintroducing foods to test your tolerance and avoid overwhelming the gut.

Daily Tasks:

- **Morning:**

    - Start with **warm water and lemon** to help detoxify your body and prepare your digestive system for food reintroduction.

    - Begin the day with a simple, easily digestible breakfast like **scrambled eggs** with spinach or a **smoothie** made with coconut milk, avocado, and a small amount of blueberries (keep it low FODMAP).

- **Meals:**

- o **Lunch:** Introduce a new food such as **zucchini noodles** or **butternut squash** (both are gentle on the gut and high in fiber).

- o **Snack:** Fresh **carrot sticks** with a small amount of almond butter (a safe, easy-to-digest snack).

- **Evening:**

  - o **Dinner: Baked chicken** with **steamed asparagus** and **quinoa** (asparagus is prebiotic and helps restore healthy gut bacteria).

  - o Have **chamomile tea** before bed for its relaxing and digestive benefits.

Key Points for Day 11:

- Reintroduce only one new food per day to monitor any potential adverse reactions.

- Focus on foods that are low FODMAP or gentle on the digestive system to minimize flare-ups.

- Keep meals simple and easy to digest to avoid overloading your gut.

Day 12: Probiotics and Prebiotics – A Balanced Approach

Focus: The significance of maintaining a balance between probiotics and prebiotics in order to support long-term recovery and nourish gut flora.

Daily Tasks:

- **Morning:**

- o Drink **water with lemon** to stimulate digestion.

- o **Probiotic Supplement:** Start incorporating **high-quality probiotics** (preferably a multi-strain formula) to help restore a healthy balance of gut bacteria.

- **Meals:**

  - o **Lunch:** Introduce fermented foods like **kimchi**, **sauerkraut**, or a small serving of **kefir** (prebiotic and probiotic-rich).

  - o **Snack:** A handful of **chia seeds** (high in fiber, omega-3s, and prebiotics) mixed into a small portion of coconut yogurt.

- **Evening:**

  - **Dinner: Grilled salmon** with a side of **cooked spinach** and **sweet potato**. Fishlike salmon provides healthy fats that support the gut lining, and spinach is rich in magnesium, which helps relax the digestive system.

  - Finish the day with a cup of **peppermint or fennel tea** to soothe your stomach and reduce any bloating.

Key Points for Day 12:

- Probiotics help replenish good bacteria, but they can sometimes cause bloating. Start with small doses and monitor your symptoms.

- Prebiotics, found in foods like garlic, onions, and certain vegetables, help feed the beneficial bacteria. Introduce them slowly and gauge your tolerance.

- Continue with gentle meals to support gut healing.

Day 13: Managing Emotional Stress and Gut Health

Focus: How stress affects your digestive system and the relationship between the stomach and the brain.

Daily Tasks:

- **Morning:**

  o Begin your day with a **relaxing mindfulness meditation** for 10 minutes to help manage stress and promote gut health.

o Have a nourishing breakfast of **oatmeal** (made with water or coconut milk) and topped with **chia seeds** and **cinnamon** (cinnamon is known for its anti-inflammatory properties).

- **Meals:**

  o **Lunch:** A light salad made with **mixed greens, avocado, grilled turkey,** and **olive oil dressing** (packed with healthy fats and protein for gut repair).

  o **Snack:** A small portion of **green apple slices** with **almond butter** (this provides fiber and healthy fats without overloading your gut).

- **Evening:**

  - Spend 15 minutes before dinner practicing **deep breathing exercises** or **progressive muscle relaxation** to help reduce cortisol levels.

  - **Dinner: Slow-cooked beef stew** with root vegetables like **carrots**, **turnips**, and **parsnips** (these are soothing, easy-to-digest vegetables).

  - Wind down with a cup of **chamomile tea** to relax and promote a restful night's sleep.

Key Points for Day 13:

- Stress can directly impact your gut health by causing inflammation and altering gut motility. Incorporating stress-reducing practices like meditation, yoga, and deep breathing is vital for healing.

- Be mindful of your emotional health—consider journaling or connecting with a support group if stress becomes overwhelming.

- Continue focusing on nourishing, easy-to-digest foods.

Day 14: Supplements for Long-Term Gut Health

Focus: Using supplements to keep the gut in balance, support it over the long run, and avoid relapses.

Daily Tasks:

- **Morning:**

o Start with **warm water** and **apple cider vinegar** to aid digestion.

o Take **probiotic supplements** (a high-quality multi-strain formula) to maintain beneficial bacteria levels.

o Add a scoop of **collagen powder** to your morning smoothie or drink to promote gut healing.

- **Meals:**

  o **Lunch:** Grilled **chicken breast** with a side of **roasted Brussels sprouts** and **quinoa**.

  o **Snack: Pumpkin seeds** (a great source of magnesium, zinc, and healthy fats) with a few **blueberries** (rich in antioxidants).

- **Evening:**

  - **Dinner:** A **green vegetable stir-fry** with **grass-fed beef, spinach, bok choy**, and **zucchini** (nutrient-dense and rich in fiber and healthy fats).

  - Enjoy a cup of **ginger tea** before bed to soothe the digestive system.

Key Points for Day 14:

- Essential supplements during this phase include probiotics, collagen, and possibly **omega-3 fatty acids** to support the gut lining.

- If your healthcare provider has recommended additional supplements like **digestive enzymes** or **magnesium**, be sure to take them as directed.

- A balanced diet rich in whole foods is crucial, but supplements can help fill in any gaps and ensure that the gut receives the necessary nutrients for long-term health.

Day 15: Reflection and Review – Assessing Your Progress

Focus: Evaluate how your body is reacting to the changes, consider your progress, and modify your healing plan as needed.

Daily Tasks:

- **Morning:**

    o **Mindful reflection**: Spend 10 minutes reflecting on how you feel—physically, emotionally, and mentally. Write down any changes in symptoms (positive or negative) and what foods/supplements have worked best.

- o **Hydration:** Drink a glass of water with a tablespoon of **lemon juice** and **cayenne pepper** (supports digestion and detoxification).

- **Meals:**

  - o **Lunch:** A light, easily digestible meal like **grilled shrimp** with a side of **avocado** and **cucumber salad**.

  - o **Snack: Coconut yogurt** with a handful of **ground flaxseeds** (rich in fiber and omega-3s).

- **Evening:**

- o **Dinner: Baked cod** with **steamed broccoli** and **cauliflower rice** (low FODMAP and gentle on the gut).

- o Wind down with **lavender tea** to help prepare for a restful sleep.

Key Points for Day 15:

- Use this day to assess how your body is responding. If you're feeling better, continue with the healing plan. If symptoms persist, consult with your healthcare provider to tweak your approach.

- Reflecting on your emotional and mental state is equally important—long-term healing is about creating a healthy relationship with food and yourself.

Key Takeaways for Days 11-15:

- **Food Reintroduction:** Begin cautiously adding foods back into your diet while monitoring your tolerance.

- **Probiotics & Prebiotics:** Focus on a balance of probiotics (good bacteria) and prebiotics (foods that feed good bacteria) to restore gut flora.

- **Stress Management:** Incorporate stress-reduction techniques like meditation, deep breathing, and journaling to reduce emotional stress, which can negatively impact gut health.

- **Supplements:** Continue using probiotics, collagen, and other supplements as needed to support gut healing and long-term gut health.

This Restoration Phase is about rebuilding and maintaining the healthy gut flora essential for long-term digestive health. By carefully reintroducing foods and focusing on lifestyle practices that nurture the gut, you can ensure that your recovery continues to progress smoothly.

Day 16-20: Maintenance Phase – Long-Term Strategies

Ensuring long-term gut health and consolidating your success are the main goals of the Maintenance Phase. Your digestive system ought to be more steady by now, and you've probably resumed eating a variety of meals without experiencing any serious problems. Creating a sustainable strategy for preserving your gut health, avoiding relapse, and making decisions that promote continued wellness is the aim of this phase.

Day 16: How to Maintain SIBO Remission

Focus: Strategies to keep SIBO symptoms under control and ensure remission is sustained.

Daily Tasks:

- **Morning:**

    - Start the day with **warm water** and **lemon juice** to alkalize your body and support digestive function.

    - **Probiotic Supplement:** Continue taking a high-quality, multi-strain **probiotic** (if not already done), which will help maintain a healthy gut microbiome.

- **Meals:**

o **Breakfast:** A nutrient-dense, easy-to-digest meal like **scrambled eggs** with **spinach** and **avocado.** Avoid excess sugar and processed foods, which can disrupt gut bacteria.

o **Lunch:** A hearty salad made with **mixed greens**, **cucumber**, **tomatoes**, **grilled chicken**, and an olive oil and **apple cider vinegar** dressing.

- **Evening:**

o **Dinner: Baked salmon** with **steamed asparagus** and **sweet potatoes.** Healthy fats from salmon and fiber from vegetables are key to gut healing.

- Enjoy a cup of **chamomile tea** or **peppermint tea** before bed to aid digestion and reduce any residual bloating.

Key Points for Day 16:

- Continue supporting your digestive system with daily probiotics to ensure a healthy gut flora.

- Aim for a **whole foods-based diet** that's rich in fiber, healthy fats, and lean proteins while avoiding processed or inflammatory foods.

- Focus on **moderate portion sizes** to avoid overwhelming your gut.

Day 17: Best Practices for Ongoing Gut Health

Focus: Developing routines that support continued digestive health and avert flare-ups in the future.

Daily Tasks:

- **Morning:**

  - Start the day with a **hydrating** drink: a glass of water with **cayenne pepper** and **lemon** to stimulate digestion.

  - Continue with **probiotic supplementation** and consider adding **prebiotics** (such as **artichokes**, **onions**, or **garlic**) into your diet to nourish beneficial bacteria.

- **Meals:**

  - **Breakfast:** A nourishing **chia pudding** made with coconut milk, chia seeds, and a handful of **blueberries**. This meal is rich in fiber and healthy fats.

  o **Lunch:** A bowl of **bone broth** with **turkey meatballs** and some **sautéed kale**. Bone broth is rich in collagen and supports gut lining integrity.

- **Evening:**

  o **Dinner: Grilled chicken** with a side of **roasted cauliflower** and **zucchini**. Cauliflower and zucchini are gut-friendly vegetables that are rich in fiber and antioxidants.

  o Before bed, enjoy a cup of **ginger tea** to help soothe any digestive discomfort and encourage relaxation.

Key Points for Day 17:

- Establish a **routine of balanced meals** that support gut health, and be mindful of food choices that may be inflammatory or gut-irritating.

- Include **digestive-supportive foods** like fermented vegetables, lean proteins, and nutrient-rich fats (avocados, coconut oil, olive oil).

- Remember that **hydration** is essential; water supports digestion and helps keep things moving in the gut.

Day 18: Identifying Triggers and Preventing Relapse

Focus: Identifying possible triggers and taking preventative action to prevent SIBO flare-ups in the future.

Daily Tasks:

- **Morning:**

  - Start with **warm water** with **apple cider vinegar** to promote digestion.

  - **Mindful Check-In:** Take a moment to check in with yourself and reflect on any symptoms you may still be experiencing. Journal about your physical, emotional, and mental state.

- **Meals:**

  - **Breakfast:** A **smoothie** made with **spinach, avocado, chia seeds**, and a scoop of **collagen powder** (helps to repair gut lining).

- o **Lunch:** A **vegetable stir-fry** with **tofu** or **chicken**, **broccoli**, **bok choy**, and **carrots**. Use **coconut oil** for cooking and a dash of **turmeric** for its anti-inflammatory properties.

- **Evening:**

  - o **Dinner: Grass-fed beef** with **roasted Brussels sprouts** and **sweet potato**. Brussels sprouts contain fiber and antioxidants that can help maintain gut health.

  - o End the evening with a **cup of peppermint tea** to help calm the digestive system before bed.

Key Points for Day 18:

- Take note of any foods or lifestyle habits that may trigger symptoms and eliminate or limit them.

- Common SIBO triggers include **high sugar intake**, **processed foods**, **dairy**, and **gluten**. Avoiding these foods can help maintain remission.

- Use **journaling** as a tool to track your food intake, stress levels, and symptoms to help identify patterns and adjust accordingly.

Day 19: Creating a Sustainable Lifestyle for Long-Term Gut Health

Focus: Developing routines that promote your general wellbeing and maintain the harmony of your digestive system.

Daily Tasks:

- **Morning:**

  - Start your day with a **hydrating drink** such as **lemon water** with a pinch of **pink Himalayan salt** to replenish electrolytes.

  - Begin with **deep breathing exercises** or a brief **meditation** to lower stress levels.

- **Meals:**

  - **Breakfast:** A bowl of **overnight oats** with **flaxseeds** and a sprinkle of **cinnamon**. Oats are soothing to the digestive tract and contain prebiotic fiber.

- Lunch: A **lentil soup** with **spinach**, **carrots**, and a squeeze of **lemon** for extra vitamin C and digestive support.

- **Evening:**

  - **Dinner: Grilled fish** (such as cod or mackerel) with a side of **steamed broccoli** and **cauliflower rice**.

  - End your day with a relaxing cup of **lavender tea** to unwind before bed.

Key Points for Day 19:

- Establish a **sustainable routine** of healthy meals, hydration, and stress management practices that you can continue long-term.

- **Mindfulness** is key to maintaining emotional health, which is closely tied to gut health. Regular relaxation practices, like yoga or meditation, will keep your stress levels in check.

Day 20: Maintaining SIBO Remission through Long-Term Lifestyle Changes

Focus: Final adjustments for long-term maintenance of gut health.

Daily Tasks:

- **Morning:**

    o Begin the day with **warm water** and **ginger** (to help with digestion and inflammation).

    o Take a moment to reflect on how far you've come. **Journal** any changes you've noticed in your symptoms or overall well-being.

- **Meals:**

  - Breakfast: **Avocado toast** on **gluten-free bread** with a sprinkle of **chia seeds**. Avocados provide healthy fats that nourish the gut.

  - **Lunch:** A balanced meal of **chicken** with **roasted vegetables** (zucchini, bell peppers, and eggplant).

- **Evening:**

  - **Dinner: Baked salmon** with a side of **sautéed greens** (spinach, kale) and **sweet potato**.

  - End with **chamomile tea** for its calming properties.

Key Points for Day 20:

- **Self-care** is an essential part of long-term gut health. Continue focusing on **mindful eating**, **stress management**, and maintaining a **regular exercise routine**.

- Continue to **avoid common triggers** (like processed foods, excessive sugar, and alcohol) to maintain remission.

- Keep adjusting your diet and lifestyle based on your body's needs to ensure that you stay on track for long-term healing.

Key Takeaways for Days 16-20:

- **SIBO Remission:** Focus on maintaining remission with a balanced, whole foods diet, and avoid foods that could trigger a relapse.

- **Long-Term Strategies:** Establish routines for **stress management**, **probiotics**,

mindful eating, and **hydration** to sustain gut health.

- **Track Progress:** Use journaling to track your symptoms, diet, and stress levels to identify any potential triggers for relapse.

Creating a sustainable lifestyle that promotes long-term gut health and solidifying the progress you've made are the goals of the Maintenance Phase. You may maintain control over SIBO and experience a long-lasting recovery by continuing to feed your body the proper foods, controlling your stress, and taking care of your physical and emotional well-being.

Day 21-25: Final Phase – Optimizing Your Gut Health

Everything you've learnt and applied throughout the earlier phases of the healing process is intended to be combined in the Final Phase. The goal of these final five days is to optimize your gut health for long-term well-being and avoid relapse by making adjustments to your food, lifestyle, and thinking. You'll learn about cutting-edge methods to improve digestion, the role that mental health plays in the healing process, and how to live a life free of SIBO going forward.

Day 21: Advanced Tips for Enhancing Digestion and Absorption

Focus: Refining your digestive system's ability to absorb nutrients and maximize healing.

Daily Tasks:

- **Morning:**

  - Start your day with **warm lemon water** to support digestion and liver detoxification.

  - Consider adding a **digestive enzyme** supplement to your routine to assist in breaking down food more efficiently, especially if you still experience any bloating or discomfort.

- **Meals:**

  - **Breakfast:** A protein-packed smoothie with **collagen peptides**, **spinach**, **frozen berries**, and a tablespoon of **flaxseed** for fiber and healthy fats. This helps keep your gut microbiome nourished and promotes proper digestion.

- **Lunch:** A **zucchini noodles** salad with **grilled shrimp**, **avocado**, and **cucumber**, topped with olive oil and **lemon dressing**. The high-water content of zucchini can support hydration and digestion.

- **Evening:**

  - **Dinner:** A meal of **grilled chicken** with a side of **roasted vegetables** (carrots, sweet potatoes, and broccoli). These vegetables are rich in fiber and antioxidants, which help support gut repair and motility.

  - Consider adding a tablespoon of **fermented food** like **kimchi** or **sauerkraut** to your meal to further encourage beneficial bacteria growth in your gut.

Key Points for Day 21:

- Digestive enzymes can facilitate digestion and aid in the absorption of nutrients, especially when returning to a more diverse diet.
- Because they support good gut flora and facilitate the digestion of more complex foods, fermented foods like kimchi, sauerkraut, and kefir are great additions to your diet.
- To avoid overtaxing your digestive system, keep eating smaller, more frequent meals.

Day 22: Mind-Body Connection: The Role of Mental Health in Healing

Focus: Understanding the profound connection between mental health and gut health, and integrating practices to support both.

Daily Tasks:

- **Morning:**
  - Start with a **morning meditation** session (10–15 minutes) to reduce stress and promote a positive mental outlook. Studies have shown that reducing stress can significantly impact gut health, as the gut-brain axis is crucial in digestion and immune function.

- **Meals:**
  - **Breakfast:** A **smoothie bowl** made with coconut milk, **chia seeds**, **avocado**, and topped with **pumpkin seeds** for extra fiber and healthy fats.

- - Lunch: A **salmon** salad with **mixed greens, cherry tomatoes**, and a **tahini dressing**. Rich in omega-3 fatty acids, salmon supports inflammation reduction, benefiting both mental and gut health.

- **Evening:**
  - - Dinner: A warm bowl of **bone broth** with **turkey meatballs** and some **cooked vegetables**. Bone broth is not only great for gut healing but also contains collagen, which has been shown to support the skin and joints.

  - - Wind-down: Practice **deep breathing** exercises or take a relaxing bath with **Epsom salts** to reduce stress and enhance overall well-being.

Key Points for Day 22:

- The **gut-brain axis** connects your emotional health to your gut health. Chronic stress or emotional distress can aggravate digestive issues, including SIBO.

- Incorporate **stress-reduction techniques** such as **yoga**, **meditation**, or **mindful breathing** into your routine to enhance gut healing and improve emotional health.

- Recognize that **mental well-being** plays a pivotal role in maintaining a healthy gut. Practicing self-care is just as important as the food you eat for long-term healing.

Day 23: Living SIBO-Free: Building a Sustainable, SIBO-Free Lifestyle

Focus: Embracing long-term strategies to prevent relapse and build a life that promotes ongoing gut health.

Daily Tasks:

- **Morning:**

  - Start your morning with a **hydrating cup of herbal tea**, such as **peppermint** or **ginger**, both of which help with digestion and soothe the stomach.

  - Begin the day with a **mindful check-in**, taking note of your physical health, emotional state, and any remaining symptoms. This will help you track progress and prevent any setbacks.

- **Meals:**

- **Breakfast:** An **avocado and egg** breakfast bowl with **spinach** and a sprinkle of **turmeric**. Avocados offer healthy fats that support gut health and reduce inflammation.

  - **Lunch:** A bowl of **lentil soup** with **spinach**, **onions**, and **carrots**. Lentils provide fiber and protein while being easily digestible.

- **Evening:**

  - **Dinner:** Grilled **turkey** with **steamed broccoli** and a side of **quinoa** for fiber and additional nutrient absorption.

  - **Evening Relaxation:** End the day with a calming **chamomile tea** to support sleep and digestion.

Key Points for Day 23:

- **Balanced meals** that focus on whole, anti-inflammatory foods are crucial for long-term gut health and preventing relapse.

- Pay attention to portion control to avoid overwhelming your digestive system and continue to practice **mindful eating** to support digestion.

- Keep in mind that **SIBO management is a lifelong commitment** to a balanced diet, good stress management, and regular lifestyle habits that support gut health.

Day 24: Preparing for Life After SIBO Recovery

Focus: Preparing yourself for a future of optimal gut health and a lifestyle that supports digestion.

Daily Tasks:

- **Morning:**

  - Begin the day with **hydrating water** infused with **cucumber** and **lemon** to keep your body refreshed.

  - Use this time for **goal-setting**, reflecting on your SIBO journey and writing down goals for maintaining your health moving forward.

- **Meals:**

  - **Breakfast:** A nourishing **green smoothie** with **spinach, chia seeds, coconut milk,** and a handful of **berries**. Packed with nutrients that support gut healing.

- o **Lunch:** A nutritious salad with **grilled chicken, avocado, mixed greens**, and **olive oil** for healthy fats.

- **Evening:**

  - o **Dinner: Baked cod** with **roasted vegetables** and a side of **wild rice** for a balanced meal rich in fiber, omega-3 fatty acids, and antioxidants.

Key Points for Day 24:

- Setting goals is crucial to sustaining a long-term healthy way of living. You'll be more likely to maintain your gut-healthy practices if you have clear aims.
- Keep in mind that maintaining a healthy lifestyle is a journey, and that having a positive outlook and specific goals can help you stay successful in living a life free of SIBO.

Day 25: Embracing a SIBO-Free Future

Focus: Celebrating your recovery and committing to a life of balance, health, and vitality.

Daily Tasks:

- **Morning:**

    o Start your final day with **water** and **apple cider vinegar** to support digestion.

    o **Reflect** on your healing process and all the progress you've made. Celebrate your achievements and your resilience.

- **Meals:**

    o **Breakfast:** A warm bowl of **oatmeal** with **flaxseed, almonds,** and **cinnamon** for a comforting, nutrient-dense start to the day.

- **Lunch:** A balanced plate of **grilled chicken, roasted Brussels sprouts**, and a side of **quinoa** for a satisfying and gut-friendly meal.

- **Evening:**

  - **Dinner: Grilled salmon** with a side of **roasted sweet potatoes** and a fresh **arugula salad**. Full of fiber, antioxidants, and omega-3s, this meal is perfect for gut health.

Key Points for Day 25:

- **Celebrate your progress**: Acknowledge how far you've come in your healing journey, and commit to maintaining your health with mindfulness and balanced nutrition.

- **Long-term success**: Your continued commitment to a **gut-healthy lifestyle** will help prevent relapse and keep you feeling your best.

Key Takeaways for Days 21-25:

- Focus on **digestive optimization** with advanced practices like probiotics, digestive enzymes, and fermented foods to improve nutrient absorption.

- Embrace the **mind-body connection** by managing stress and maintaining emotional health, which are essential for sustaining a healthy gut.

- Build a **SIBO-free lifestyle** by incorporating balanced meals, staying mindful of triggers, and continuing habits that promote optimal gut health for the long term.

With these final steps, you'll be well on your way
to a life free from the discomforts of SIB

Chapter 5

Supplementation and Alternative Treatments

When it comes to treating Small Intestinal Bacterial Overgrowth (SIBO), a comprehensive method that includes dietary adjustments, lifestyle changes, and targeted treatments can greatly enhance your chances of recovery.

While diet plays a foundational part in healing, the use of supplements and alternative treatments can support your body's natural healing processes, help restore balance in the gut microbiome, and address underlying issues that contribute to SIBO.

In this chapter, we'll explore the best supplements for SIBO, herbal remedies, natural treatments, and the use of antibiotics and prokinetics—all important components in a holistic SIBO recovery plan.

Best Supplements for SIBO

Certain supplements can provide significant support during the healing process, especially when used alongside dietary and lifestyle changes.

These supplements can address imbalances in gut flora, lower inflammation, improve digestion, and support general gut health. Here's a breakdown of the most helpful supplements for SIBO recovery:

1. Probiotics

Probiotics are live helpful bacteria that can help restore a healthy balance of gut flora. While the use of probiotics in SIBO treatment is somewhat controversial—especially during the initial stages when bacterial overgrowth is present—probiotics can be helpful in the restoration phase (Day 11-15) when you begin rebuilding your gut flora. Specific strains such as Lactobacillus and Bifidobacterium can help repopulate the gut with good bacteria and improve digestive health.

Benefits:

- Helps restore balance in the gut bacteria.
- Reduces gut inflammation and improves digestion.
- May lower gas production and bloating by supporting healthy gut flora.

Caution:

Probiotics should be used carefully during the early phases of SIBO treatment, as introducing too many bacteria may exacerbate symptoms. Always consult with a healthcare source before adding probiotics to your regimen.

2. Digestive Enzymes

Digestive enzymes help break down food more effectively, which can be particularly helpful in cases of SIBO, where the overgrowth of bacteria impairs nutrient absorption. These enzymes help prevent undigested food from fermenting in the small intestine, which can lead to bloating, gas, and discomfort.

Benefits:

- Assists in the digestion of carbs, fats, and proteins.
- Supports nutrient intake, preventing deficiencies.
- Can reduce bloating and pain after meals.

Common Enzymes:

- Amylase (for carbohydrates), lipase (for fats), and protease (for proteins).

3. L-Glutamine

L-glutamine is an amino acid that plays a key role in gut healing. It supports the intestinal lining, reduces intestinal permeability (also known as leaky gut), and helps in the repair of the mucosal barrier. This supplement is particularly useful in restoring gut health, especially after months or years of digestive dysfunction.

Benefits:

- Helps repair the gut walls and reduces inflammation.
- Improves gut barrier function and stops leaky gut.
- Supports general digestive health and immune function.

4. Berberine

Berberine is a powerful plant compound with antimicrobial qualities. It has been shown to help control bacterial overgrowth and improve insulin sensitivity, which is important for general metabolic health. Some studies show berberine can help restore balance in the gut microbiome by inhibiting pathogenic bacteria and promoting beneficial bacteria growth.

Benefits:

- Supports gut microbial balance by inhibiting harmful bugs.
- Helps reduce intestinal inflammation and support gut health.
- Can help in blood sugar regulation, supporting metabolic health.

5. Zinc Carnosine

Zinc carnosine is a mixture of zinc and the amino acid carnosine. This supplement has been shown to support the healing of the gut lining, lower inflammation, and improve the function of the small intestine. It is particularly helpful for individuals with leaky gut or other digestive problems that compromise the intestinal barrier.

Benefits:

- Promotes gut lining repair and integrity.
- Reduces symptoms of intestinal permeability.
- Supports immune health and general gut function.

Herbal Remedies and Natural Treatments

In addition to supplements, many people with SIBO turn to herbal remedies and natural treatments to support healing. Herbal remedies can help lower inflammation, kill harmful bacteria, and improve digestion. Here are some widely used herbs and natural treatments for SIBO:

1. Oregano Oil

Oregano oil is a powerful antimicrobial herb that can help kill harmful bacteria in the small intestine. It is particularly effective against certain types of bacteria linked with SIBO, especially gram-negative bacteria. Oregano oil has natural antibacterial, antifungal, and antiviral effects.

Benefits:

- Helps remove harmful bacteria in the gut.
- Reduces inflammation and helps gut health.
- May improve gut movement and digestion.

Usage:

Oregano oil should be used with care and in proper dosage, as it is highly concentrated. Consult with a healthcare provider before using oregano oil, especially if you're also taking antibiotics.

2. Garlic Extract

Garlic is another powerful natural antimicrobial that has been shown to help reduce bacterial overgrowth in the small intestine. Allicin, the active compound in garlic, has antibacterial, antifungal, and antiviral benefits.

Benefits:

- Supports the elimination of harmful bacteria.
- Reduces gas, bloating, and inflammation.
- Boosts immune system function and general digestive health.

Usage:

Garlic extract can be used in supplement form or as part of your food. Garlic may be too strong for some people and could lead to digestive discomfort, so start with small doses.

3. Peppermint Oil

Peppermint oil is known for its ability to soothe the digestive system and improve motility. It has been found to lessen symptoms such as bloating, gas, and cramping by relaxing the muscles in the intestines and promoting better digestion.

Benefits:

- Relieves abdominal discomfort and cramping.
- Supports motility and smooth muscle action in the intestines.
- Reduces bloating and gas production.

Usage:

Peppermint oil is often used in enteric-coated capsules to ensure it enters the intestines without causing irritation in the stomach.

4. Ginger

Ginger is another herb with anti-inflammatory and stomach benefits. It helps stimulate digestion, soothe nausea, and reduce inflammation in the digestive system. Ginger can also increase gut motility, which is important for SIBO treatment.

Benefits:

- Supports digestion and reduces nausea.
- Stimulates movement, helping prevent bacterial overgrowth.
- Reduces inflammation and soothes the digestive system.

Usage:

Fresh ginger, ginger tea, or ginger supplements can be added to your daily routine to support gut health.

The Role of Antibiotics and Prokinetics in SIBO Treatment

In many cases, antibiotics and prokinetics (medications that improve gut motility) are essential parts of SIBO treatment. Both can help address the root causes of SIBO and avoid relapse.

1. Antibiotics for SIBO

Antibiotics are often recommended to target the overgrowth of harmful bacteria in the small intestine. The two most widely used antibiotics for SIBO treatment are rifaximin and neomycin.

- **Rifaximin:**

This is a broad-spectrum antibiotic that targets the gut bacteria. It has been shown to lower the number of bacteria in the small intestine without disrupting the balance of bacteria in the large intestine. Rifaximin is usually used for hydrogen SIBO.

- **Neomycin:**

Neomycin is often used to treat methane-producing SIBO caused by methanobrevibacter smithii. Methane is produced by archaea (not bacteria), and neomycin is useful against these organisms.

Benefits:

- Helps remove harmful bacteria in the small intestine.
- Can greatly reduce symptoms like bloating, pain, and diarrhea.

Caution:

Antibiotics should only be used under the direction of a healthcare provider, as overuse can lead to antibiotic resistance and disrupt gut flora.

2. Prokinetics

Prokinetics are medicines that help restore proper motility in the gut. Many people with SIBO also have intestinal motility problems, which can make it difficult for the small intestine to move food and waste properly, creating an environment where bacteria can overgrow.

Common Prokinetics:

- Low-dose naltrexone (LDN): Used to improve gut motility and reduce inflammation.
- Erythromycin: An antibiotic that can be used at low doses to help increase gut motility.

- Motegrity (prucalopride): A medication especially designed to improve motility in the intestines.

Benefits:

- Helps restore normal gut motility and avoid bacterial overgrowth.
- Reduces constipation and improves general digestive function.

Caution:

Prokinetics should only be used under medical supervision, especially if you have underlying conditions affecting motility or other health issues.

Key Takeaways

- Supplements like probiotics, digestive enzymes, L-glutamine, berberine, and zinc carnosine can support healing by restoring gut integrity, lowering inflammation, and balancing gut flora.

- Herbal remedies such as oregano oil, garlic, peppermint oil, and ginger can help in reducing bacterial overgrowth, soothing digestive discomfort, and improving motility.

- Antibiotics and prokinetics play a vital part in the treatment of SIBO by targeting bacterial overgrowth and improving gut motility.

By integrating the right mix of supplements, herbal treatments, and medications into your SIBO recovery plan, you can optimize your gut health and move towards long-term remission. However, always consult with a healthcare professional before starting any new supplements or treatments to ensure that they are appropriate for your individual needs.

Chapter 6

Lifestyle Factors and SIBO

When it comes to healing from Small Intestinal Bacterial Overgrowth (SIBO), lifestyle factors play a crucial part. While diet and supplementation are important for addressing the bacterial overgrowth directly, how you manage stress, sleep, and physical activity can have a profound effect on your gut health and overall recovery. In this chapter, we'll explore how stress management, sleep, and exercise influence your digestive system and SIBO healing, giving practical tips to help you optimize these areas for better health.

Stress Management: Techniques for Healing

Chronic stress is one of the most significant factors leading to gut dysbiosis, or an imbalance in your gut bacteria. When you're worried, your body goes into "fight or flight" mode, releasing hormones like cortisol that can negatively affect digestion and immune function.

This can increase SIBO symptoms by slowing down gut motility, making it easier for bacteria to overgrow. Additionally, stress can contribute to increased intestinal permeability, widely known as leaky gut, which can make it harder for your body to heal.

Why Stress Matters for SIBO:

1. *Slows digestion:* When under stress, blood is redirected away from the digestive system to support other processes, leading to slower digestion and promoting bacterial overgrowth.

2. *Disrupts gut motility:* Stress can impair the normal contractions of the intestines, resulting in constipation or poor food transit, providing a perfect environment for bacterial overgrowth.

3. *Weakens the immune system:* Chronic stress suppresses your immune function, which is important to control harmful bacteria in the gut.

Stress Management Techniques:

1. *Mindfulness Meditation* – Practicing mindfulness Meditation for just 10-15 minutes a day can help lower cortisol levels and improve gut health by calming the nervous system. Meditation helps you stay present and reduce the mental load that adds to stress.

2. *Deep Breathing Exercises* – Focused breathing methods, such as diaphragmatic breathing, activate the parasympathetic nervous system, which is responsible for "rest and digest." This helps to relax the digestive system, improving motility and lowering stress on the gut.

3. *Yoga and Stretching* – Gentle yoga stretches can help activate the vagus nerve, a key component in regulating digestion. Yoga also improves circulation to the gut, encouraging better digestive function and reducing bloating and pain.

4. *Cognitive Behavioral Therapy (CBT)* – If stress or anxiety is chronic, CBT can help you create healthier thought patterns and coping strategies. Working with a therapist can be helpful for managing stress linked to digestive health.

5. *Nature Walks* – Taking time to walk in nature can help reduce cortisol levels and improve general well-being. A short walk after meals can also aid digestion and prevent post-meal bloating.

How Sleep Affects Your Gut Health

Sleep is a cornerstone of overall health, and its connection with gut health cannot be overstated. Poor or insufficient sleep can impair digestion, disrupt gut flora balance, and increase your sensitivity to conditions like SIBO. During sleep, your body enters a restorative phase that helps control immune function, repair tissues, and support the balance of beneficial bacteria in the gut.

Why Sleep Matters for SIBO:

1. Supports digestion and repair: During deep sleep, the body prioritizes repair and renewal, including the restoration of the gut lining. Adequate sleep is important for maintaining a healthy intestinal barrier, preventing leaky gut, and allowing your digestive system to work optimally.

2. Regulates the gut-brain axis: The gut and brain are closely related through the gut-brain axis. Poor sleep increases stress and can disrupt this connection, leading to worsened digestive problems and SIBO symptoms.

3. Influences microbiome diversity: Studies show that sleep deprivation can change the composition of your gut microbiome, favoring the growth of harmful bacteria over beneficial ones. This imbalance can exacerbate SIBO symptoms.

How to Improve Sleep for Gut Health:

1. *Establish a Regular Sleep Schedule* – Try to go to bed and wake up at the same time every day to control your body's circadian rhythm. Consistent sleep patterns help support restorative sleep.

2. *Create a Relaxing Bedtime Routine* – Engage in calming activities such as reading, writing, or taking a warm bath before bed to signal to your body that it's time to wind down. Avoid screens (phones, computers, TVs) at least 30 minutes before bedtime, as blue light can interfere with melatonin production.

3. *Limit Stimulants* – Avoid coffee, nicotine, and heavy meals close to bedtime. These drugs can interfere with your ability to fall asleep and disrupt the quality of your rest.

4. Create an Optimal Sleep Environment –
Keep your bedroom cool, dark, and quiet to support deep, restorative sleep. Invest in a comfortable mattress and pillows that support good balance throughout the night.

5. Manage Nighttime Stress – If stress or anxiety keeps you awake, try a relaxation method before bed, such as deep breathing or progressive muscle relaxation. Journaling before bed can also help you unload your thoughts and clear your mind.

The Importance of Regular Exercise for Digestion

Exercise isn't just good for your heart and muscles; it plays an important role in your gut health as well. Physical exercise helps to stimulate the motility of the intestines, encouraging the movement of food through your digestive system and preventing stagnation, which can contribute to bacterial overgrowth. Regular exercise has also been shown to have a positive effect on the diversity and balance of gut microbiota, which is crucial for avoiding and managing conditions like SIBO.

Why Exercise Matters for SIBO:

1. *Improves gut motility:* Exercise helps stimulate the muscles of the digestive system, encouraging the movement of food and waste through the intestines. This reduces the chance of bacterial overgrowth, especially in the small intestine, and improves overall digestive function.

2. *Reduces bloating and constipation:* Physical exercise promotes regular bowel movements and can reduce symptoms of bloating and constipation, which are common in individuals with SIBO.

3. *Promotes a healthy microbiome:* Studies show that regular physical activity enhances microbial diversity in the gut. A balanced microbiome is key to avoiding the conditions that lead to SIBO.

4. *Boosts immune function:* Exercise helps improve immune system function, which is important for controlling the overgrowth of harmful bacteria in the gut.

Exercise Tips for SIBO Recovery:

1. *Start Slowly and Build Gradually* – If you're new to exercise or have been idle for some time, start with light activities such as walking or gentle stretching. Gradually increase the intensity as your body changes.

2. *Aim for Consistency* – Try to incorporate moderate exercise into your daily practice. Aim for at least 30 minutes of moderate-intensity exercise, such as brisk walking, cycling, or swimming, most days of the week.

3. *Focus on Low-Impact Exercise* – High-intensity workouts or excessive cardio can put stress on the body, possibly exacerbating SIBO symptoms. Focus on low-impact workouts like walking, yoga, Pilates, or swimming to improve digestion without overtaxing the body.

4. *Incorporate Post-Meal Movement* – A short walk after meals can help stimulate digestion and avoid post-meal bloating. Even light movement helps your intestines handle food more efficiently.

5. *Listen to Your Body* – While exercise is important for gut health, be aware of how your body responds. If intense exercise causes symptoms like bloating or fatigue, scale back and focus on gentler forms of movement.

Key Takeaways:

- **Stress management** is important for healing from SIBO. Techniques like mindfulness, yoga, and deep breathing can help reduce stress hormones, improve gut motility, and support general digestive health.
- **Sleep** is important for gut repair and the restoration of the gut microbiome. A consistent sleep schedule and a calming nighttime routine can enhance the quality of your rest and support healing.

- Regular **exercise** supports **digestion** by improving gut motility, reducing bloating and constipation, and boosting general immune function. Focus on low-impact, consistent tasks that are gentle on the body during recovery.

By addressing these lifestyle factors—stress, sleep, and exercise—you can greatly enhance your healing process and improve your chances of long-term SIBO remission.

Chapter 7

Common Myths and Misunderstandings About SIBO

SIBO (Small Intestinal Bacterial Overgrowth) can be a challenging condition to handle. Between the different treatments, dietary recommendations, and the confusing range of symptoms, it's easy to become overwhelmed or misinformed.

Over the years, several myths and misconceptions about SIBO have emerged, causing confusion about its causes, diagnosis, and treatment.

In this chapter, we'll explore some of the most common myths about SIBO, disprove them with current knowledge, and provide clarity on what you really need to understand to successfully heal from this condition.

Dispelling the Most Common SIBO Myths

1. Myth 1: SIBO Is Just Another Case of IBS (Irritable Bowel Syndrome)

While SIBO and IBS share similar symptoms, they are not the same disease. IBS is a functional gastrointestinal disease that affects bowel motility and causes symptoms like diarrhea, constipation, and abdominal pain. On the other hand, SIBO is defined by an overgrowth of bacteria in the small intestine, which interferes with digestion and nutrient absorption.

Though both conditions may overlap, such as in patients with IBS having bloating or diarrhea,

SIBO is a treatable underlying condition that can sometimes be mistaken for IBS.

Reality: SIBO is a treatable condition, and identifying it as the root cause of symptoms like bloating, abdominal pain, and fatigue is important for proper treatment. Diagnosing and treating SIBO often includes different approaches than treating IBS.

2. Myth 2: SIBO Only Affects People With Digestive Disorders

Although SIBO is more often associated with digestive disorders like irritable bowel syndrome (IBS), Crohn's disease, or celiac disease, it can affect anyone. Factors such as a weakened immune system, past gastrointestinal surgeries, poor food, chronic stress, or lifestyle factors can all contribute to the development of SIBO. It is a common misconception that you have to have a pre-existing digestive disease to develop SIBO.

Reality: SIBO can form in anyone, even those without a prior history of digestive issues. Understanding that many lifestyle factors contribute to the development of SIBO is important for prevention and treatment.

3. **Myth 3: SIBO Can Be Cured with Antibiotics Alone**

While antibiotics, especially rifaximin, are a common and effective treatment for SIBO, they are not a permanent solution. Antibiotics can help lower bacterial overgrowth in the small intestine, but they don't address the underlying factors that cause SIBO in the first place. Without treating issues like diet, motility problems, or stress, SIBO can return after treatment.

Reality: Antibiotics are just one part of the healing plan. Long-term recovery from SIBO requires a holistic approach, including food modifications, lifestyle changes, and sometimes supplementation. A comprehensive plan is important for keeping remission and preventing relapse.

4. Myth 4: SIBO Is Only About Diet – If You Eat the Right Foods, It Will Go Away

Diet plays a major role in managing SIBO, but it's not the only factor. While a Low FODMAP diet, Specific Carbohydrate Diet (SCD), or elemental diet can help reduce symptoms by removing foods that feed harmful bacteria, these approaches do not necessarily remove the root causes of SIBO.

Factors like intestinal motility problems, gut bacteria imbalances, and underlying medical conditions also play important roles in the development and recurrence of SIBO.

Reality: A healthy diet is important, but a holistic approach is needed for long-term healing. Addressing underlying causes, such as gut motility, stress, and immune system function, is important for preventing a relapse of SIBO.

5. **Myth 5: SIBO Is Not a Serious Condition – It's Just a Digestive Problem**

SIBO can lead to major health complications if left untreated. Because of the bacterial overgrowth, nutrient malabsorption is common, leading to deficiencies in important vitamins and minerals, such as vitamin B12, iron, and vitamin D.

Additionally, untreated SIBO can cause chronic fatigue, unexplained weight loss, brain fog, and even intestinal permeability (leaky gut), which can lead to more serious autoimmune and inflammatory conditions.

Reality: SIBO is a serious condition that can impact your general health, especially if left untreated. It's important to take symptoms carefully and seek proper diagnosis and treatment.

Debunking Misconceptions About Diets and Treatments

1. **Myth 6: The Low FODMAP Diet is a Permanent Solution for SIBO**

The Low FODMAP diet is often given to people with SIBO to help manage symptoms. However, it's important to remember that this diet is not a cure for SIBO. It is meant to be used as a short-term strategy to lessen symptoms by eliminating certain foods that ferment in the gut. Following the Low FODMAP diet long-term can possibly deprive you of important nutrients, as it eliminates many fruits, vegetables, and whole grains that are essential for a balanced diet.

Reality: The Low FODMAP diet is a tool to manage symptoms, but it is not a lifelong solution. Once symptoms have been controlled, a phase of reintroducing foods should be followed under the direction of a healthcare provider to restore nutrient balance and improve gut health.

2. Myth 7: Probiotics Are Always Good for SIBO

Probiotics are often touted as a great supplement for improving gut health, but they are not always helpful for people with SIBO. Since SIBO is marked by overgrowth of bacteria in the small intestine, taking probiotics (which contain beneficial bacteria) can sometimes make symptoms worse, especially in the early stages of treatment. For some people with SIBO, adding probiotics too early can cause bloating, gas, or discomfort as it may feed the existing bacteria.

Reality: While probiotics can play a role in restoring a healthy gut flora balance, they should be given carefully and at the right time in the healing process. It's important to work with a healthcare provider to decide if probiotics are appropriate and when to start using them.

3. Myth 8: Once You Treat SIBO, You're Done – It Won't Come Back

While SIBO can be treated successfully, it has a tendency to recur if the underlying causes are not addressed. This can include poor gut motility, imbalances in gut bacteria, or lifestyle factors such as chronic stress or poor food. Some people may find that their symptoms return after finishing treatment, especially if they haven't made sustainable changes to their lifestyle or diet.

Reality: SIBO can return if the underlying factors are not handled. Long-term gut health maintenance includes a holistic approach, including a balanced diet, stress management, and regular monitoring by a healthcare provider.

4. Myth 9: A Low-Carb or Gluten-Free Diet Will Always Heal SIBO

While certain dietary changes can help handle SIBO symptoms, no one-size-fits-all diet works for everyone. A low-carb diet or gluten-free diet might help some people, but they are not the only dietary methods to SIBO. Diets like the Specific Carbohydrate Diet (SCD), elemental diets, or Low FODMAP diet have also shown success in managing symptoms and improving gut health. It's important to remember that what works for one person may not work for another.

Reality: There is no single "magic" food for SIBO. Diet plans should be tailored to each individual's needs, based on their symptoms, SIBO type, and general health condition.

Key Takeaways:

- SIBO is not the same as IBS. While symptoms can overlap, it's important to differentiate between these conditions for proper treatment.

- SIBO can affect anyone. It's not limited to those with pre-existing digestive issues, and many factors can add to its development.

- Diet alone is not enough. SIBO treatment needs a comprehensive approach, including addressing underlying causes and lifestyle factors.

- Antibiotics and diet adjustments are required but not sufficient for long-term healing. Treatment needs a holistic approach and long-term lifestyle changes to keep remission.

- Myths about probiotics, diet, and treatments can lead to misunderstanding. Be educated, and work with your healthcare provider to develop a personalized plan that supports your healing.

By understanding these myths and misconceptions, you'll be better equipped to manage your SIBO recovery with clarity, avoiding common pitfalls and staying on track toward healing.

Chapter 8

How to Work with Your Healthcare Provider

When dealing with SIBO, one of the most important factors for successful recovery is collaborating effectively with your healthcare provider. The road to healing from SIBO can be complicated, and having a supportive and knowledgeable medical team can make all the difference.

Whether you're working with a gastroenterologist, a functional medicine doctor, or a nutritionist, your relationship with your healthcare provider should be one of teamwork and mutual understanding. In this chapter, we'll explore how to work together with your healthcare provider for the best outcomes, understand your lab results and diagnosis, and navigate treatment options successfully.

Collaborating with a Doctor on Your Healing Journey

The first step in healing from SIBO is having a strong, communicative relationship with your healthcare provider. Here's how to approach this partnership:

1. Be Open and Honest About Your Symptoms:

It's important to share as much detail as possible about your symptoms, including the onset, duration, severity, and any triggers you've noticed. Symptoms like bloating, diarrhea, constipation, tiredness, and brain fog are often common in SIBO, but they can also overlap with other conditions. Be as detailed as possible when describing how your symptoms affect your day-to-day life.

2. Ask for a Comprehensive Evaluation:

Your healthcare provider should take a full medical history, including any gastrointestinal issues, surgeries, or conditions that may contribute to SIBO. They should also ask about your lifestyle habits, stress levels, and any medications you're taking. This will help your doctor discover potential underlying causes of your SIBO and tailor your treatment plan accordingly.

3. fight for Testing:

Many people with SIBO have to fight for proper testing. Standard tests include breath tests (like the lactulose and glucose breath tests) to identify bacterial overgrowth. If your doctor isn't suggesting these tests, it's okay to ask for them. Also, ask about other diagnostic procedures such as stool tests or small intestine imaging, which can help measure the state of your gut.

4. Be Informed:

Educate yourself about SIBO. The more you know, the better ready you'll be to have informed discussions with your healthcare provider. This can also help you feel more confident in understanding your treatment plan and the reasoning behind your doctor's suggestions.

5. Work Together on a Personalized Treatment Plan:

Every patient with SIBO is different, so treatment plans should be personalized. Your healthcare provider may suggest a mix of antibiotics, dietary changes, probiotics, and lifestyle interventions. Be sure to share any preferences or concerns you have, including your comfort level with certain treatments (e.g., using antibiotics versus natural remedies).

6. Follow Up Regularly:

SIBO recovery can take time, so be sure to plan regular follow-up appointments to monitor your progress. If your symptoms continue or worsen, don't hesitate to reach out to your doctor. Treatment may need to be adjusted along the way based on how you're reacting.

Understanding Lab Results and Diagnosis

One of the biggest hurdles in treating SIBO is knowing the results of your tests. Since many of the symptoms of **SIBO** overlap with other digestive diseases, diagnosis can be tricky. Here's how to navigate your test results:

1. Breath Test Results:

The lactulose breath test and glucose breath test are the most popular ways to diagnose **SIBO**. Both tests measure the gases released by the bacteria in the small intestine when they ferment undigested sugars.

a. Hydrogen and Methane Levels: Elevated levels of hydrogen or methane in your breath suggest an overgrowth of bacteria in the small intestine. Hydrogen is usually associated with diarrhea-predominant SIBO, while methane is linked to constipation-predominant **SIBO**.

b. Interpretation: High amounts of these gases in your breath at specific time intervals suggest that

SIBO is present. The exact threshold for a positive result may vary slightly based on the test and lab, so it's important to discuss these values with your doctor.

2. Stool Tests:

Stool tests can help identify markers of intestinal permeability (leaky gut), inflammation, and dysbiosis (an imbalance of gut bacteria), which are often linked with **SIBO**. While not the main diagnostic tool for SIBO, stool tests can provide additional information about your gut health and help guide treatment.

3. Imaging and Endoscopy:

In certain cases, imaging tests such as CT scans or upper GI endoscopy may be needed to rule out other diseases like Crohn's disease, gastroparesis (slow gastric emptying), or structural abnormalities in the intestines. Your doctor will guide you on whether these tests are necessary.

4. Interpreting Your Results:

Once your tests are complete, your doctor will interpret the results to confirm whether you have **SIBO** and decide which type (hydrogen, methane, or mixed). It's important to understand that no single test is perfect; false negatives or positives can occur, so your doctor may look at your clinical symptoms alongside lab results to make a complete diagnosis.

Navigating Treatment Options: What to Ask Your Doctor

Once you have a diagnosis, it's time to discuss treatment choices. Here are some key questions to ask your healthcare provider to ensure that you understand the treatment plan and are happy with it:

1. *What Type of SIBO Do I Have?*

Knowing whether you have hydrogen-dominant, methane-dominant, or mixed **SIBO** is important for tailoring your treatment. Different types of **SIBO** may react better to certain treatments, such as specific antibiotics, dietary changes, or even probiotics.

2. *What Are My Treatment Options?*

Discuss the various treatment options offered, which may include:

a. Antibiotics: The most typically prescribed antibiotics for SIBO are rifaximin (for hydrogen SIBO) and neomycin or metronidazole (for methane SIBO). Ask about possible side effects and the duration of treatment.

b. Herbal Antibiotics: If you prefer a more natural approach, herbal antimicrobials such as oregano oil, berberine, or garlic extract might be suggested. Inquire about the effectiveness and safety of these choices.

c. Prokinetics: To address motility issues (which often contribute to SIBO), your doctor may suggest prokinetic medications like low-dose naltrexone (LDN), prucalopride, or erythromycin to help stimulate intestinal movement.

d. Dietary Interventions: Diet is a cornerstone of SIBO treatment. Ask your doctor about specific dietary protocols like the Low FODMAP diet, Specific Carbohydrate Diet (SCD), or an elemental diet, and what might work best for your particular case.

3. What Role Do Probiotics Play in My Treatment?

Probiotics can be controversial in SIBO treatment, as adding them too early can sometimes worsen symptoms. Ask your doctor when it might be acceptable to start probiotics and which strains might be helpful (e.g., Lactobacillus and Bifidobacterium). The timing of introducing probiotics should be based on your recovery process.

4. How Will My Progress Be Monitored?

Discuss how often you should have follow-up visits to watch your symptoms and whether additional tests (such as another breath test) will be needed.

Keep in mind that treatment might need to be adjusted based on your reaction to therapy.

5. What Are the Risks of Recurrence, and How Can I Prevent It?

SIBO has a tendency to return, so it's important to ask your doctor how to keep long-term remission. Ask about lifestyle changes (such as stress management and exercise) and dietary adjustments that can help avoid a relapse of bacterial overgrowth.

Working with your healthcare provider is crucial to completely healing from SIBO. By encouraging open communication, advocating for proper testing, understanding your lab results, and knowing the treatment options available, you'll be able to manage your healing journey with confidence.

Remember that SIBO recovery is often a long-term process, requiring patience, determination, and a collaborative effort between you and your healthcare provider.

The better you understand your condition and treatment plan, the more confident you will feel in your journey toward better digestive health.

Chapter 9

Real-Life Success Stories

One of the most powerful ways to inspire and empower yourself on your SIBO healing journey is by hearing from others who have faced similar battles and found success. In this chapter, we'll share personal accounts of individuals who have battled SIBO, overcome its difficulties, and regained their health. These stories offer not just hope, but also useful insights and practical tips that you can incorporate into your own recovery plan.

Personal Accounts of Overcoming SIBO

1. Sarah's Journey: From Bloating to Balance Sarah, a 34-year-old marketing executive, had been struggling with digestive problems for over five years. Chronic bloating, cramping, and fatigue had become a part of her daily life, despite countless doctor trips and a range of treatments. She was diagnosed with SIBO after a breath test showed elevated hydrogen levels, suggesting bacterial overgrowth in her small intestine. Initially overwhelmed, Sarah felt like she had hit a breaking point.

"Every meal felt like a gamble," she says. "I never knew if I'd be bloated or in pain, or worse—running to the bathroom."

But after starting a mix of antibiotics, a Low FODMAP diet, and probiotics, Sarah began to notice changes. Slowly, the bloating eased, her energy levels improved, and she was able to enjoy food again without constant discomfort. After months of care, Sarah was in remission and living symptom-free.

Sarah's Key Takeaways:

- *Diet is critical:* The Low FODMAP diet was a game-changer for me. Cutting out foods that were irritating my gut helped greatly in reducing bloating and other symptoms.
- *Patience is key:* Recovery wasn't fast. It took several months to notice a major improvement, but I stuck with the plan.
- *Stress control matters:* Reducing stress was a huge part of my healing. Meditation and taking

time to relax helped my gut and my general well-being.

2. *James' Story:* Battling Methane SIBO James, a 40-year-old father of two, had battled with constipation for most of his adult life. It wasn't until he began suffering severe bloating, fatigue, and brain fog that he sought medical help. After a breath test showed methane SIBO, James started a tailored treatment plan that combined rifaximin, neomycin (to target methane-producing bacteria), and lifestyle changes.

"I had no idea SIBO could affect your mind so much," James says. "I felt like I was in a fog all the time, and I couldn't focus at work or at home."

For James, controlling his SIBO was a long process. The antibiotics helped lower the methane-producing bacteria, but it wasn't just about medication. He also worked closely with a dietitian to adopt the Specific Carbohydrate Diet (SCD), which helped reduce inflammation and support gut healing.

"Probiotics were a huge part of my recovery, too," he shares. "I introduced them slowly, and they made a noticeable difference in my digestion and gut flora."

James' Key Takeaways:

- Antibiotics and food together: For methane SIBO, a mix of antibiotics and the Specific Carbohydrate Diet worked best. It wasn't just about killing bacteria—it was about healing my gut walls.
- Start slow with probiotics: Probiotics were tricky at first, but once I found the right types

for me, they made a big difference in my gut health.

- Listen to your body: If something isn't working, don't hesitate to share it with your doctor. I had to change my treatment plan a few times, and that was okay.

3. *Rachel's Experience: Healing with a Holistic Approach*

Rachel, a 29-year-old yoga teacher, found her way to a SIBO diagnosis after months of digestive turmoil, including bloating, nausea, and a feeling of fullness after eating small amounts of food. Her breath test showed high levels of hydrogen, and her doctor suggested a course of rifaximin along with a strict Low FODMAP diet.

However, Rachel wanted to try a more holistic approach to healing. Alongside the medical treatment, she began working with a nutritionist who stressed gut-healing foods, such as bone broth, fermented vegetables, and anti-inflammatory herbs like turmeric and ginger. She also took up mindfulness practices like meditation and yoga to help manage the stress that was adding to her digestive problems.

"The combination of modern medicine and holistic practices was life-changing," Rachel says. "Not only did my digestion improve, but I felt more in tune with my body."

Rachel's holistic approach to healing allowed her to reintroduce foods slowly and carefully, learning how her body reacted and changing her diet accordingly. Within six months, she was free of symptoms and had returned her energy.

Key Takeaways:

- Holistic healing: Combining conventional treatments like antibiotics with holistic practices (e.g., yoga, mindfulness, and gut-healing foods) sped my recovery.

- Diet reintroduction is gradual: I took my time reintroducing foods. It wasn't a race, and I had to listen carefully to how my body reacted.

- Mind-body connection: Healing isn't just physical. Managing stress through practices like yoga and meditation played a key role in my overall recovery.

Tips and Insights from Those Who've Healed

1. Be Consistent with Your Treatment Plan

Success doesn't come overnight. One of the most popular pieces of advice from those who have healed from SIBO is to stick with your treatment plan. Whether it's antibiotics, food changes, or probiotics, consistency is key. Your gut needs time to heal, and it's important to stay committed to the plan even when progress seems slow.

2. Work Closely with Your Healthcare Team

Healing from SIBO often takes a team approach. Whether it's your doctor, a nutritionist, or a holistic health practitioner, having a team you trust can help guide you through the ups and downs of healing. Don't hesitate to ask questions, share concerns, or request additional testing if things don't feel right.

3. Track Your Symptoms and Progress

Keeping a record of your symptoms, food intake, and any changes you notice can help you track your recovery. This is especially helpful for replacing foods. It also gives you important insights into which foods or treatments work best for your unique case of SIBO.

4. Don't Be Afraid to Experiment (with Guidance)

While it's important to follow your healthcare provider's advice, many people find success by experimenting with different diets, supplements, or even stress-reduction methods. As long as you're led by a professional, it's okay to make adjustments along the way.

5. Patience and Persistence Are Key

Healing from SIBO can take time. It's not unusual to feel discouraged during the recovery process, especially if symptoms persist or flare up. However, perseverance is important. Most people who have healed from SIBO stress the importance of patience—your body needs time to rebalance, and it's okay to take it step by step.

6. Celebrate Small Wins

As you improve in your recovery, take time to celebrate the small wins. Whether it's a day without bloating, a successful food reintroduction, or an improvement in your energy levels, recognizing these milestones can keep you inspired and focused on your healing journey.

The stories shared in this part offer real-life inspiration for anyone dealing with SIBO. Although each person's path to healing is different, the common themes of perseverance, consistency, and a holistic approach to recovery are obvious. By learning from others who have healed, you can find hope, motivation, and valuable insights that will help you on your own road to reclaim your gut health. Remember, you are not alone in this, and with the right treatment plan and mindset, healing from SIBO is entirely possible.

Conclusion

Healing from Small Intestinal Bacterial Overgrowth (SIBO) is a challenging yet totally achievable journey. Throughout this book, we've explored every facet of SIBO—from knowing the science behind it to practical steps for recovery, and real-life success stories that highlight the resilience and persistence of those who have overcome it.

Whether you're newly diagnosed or have been living with SIBO for years, the roadmap given here is meant to guide you through the complexities of treatment, diet, and lifestyle changes with clarity and actionable strategies.

What we've learned:

Understanding SIBO is the foundation of any good treatment plan. Recognizing the symptoms, types, and underlying causes of SIBO equips you with the knowledge to make informed choices about your health.

Diet plays a key role in managing and recovering from SIBO. Choosing the right foods to heal your gut, while avoiding those that exacerbate symptoms, is important for reducing inflammation, balancing gut bacteria, and improving digestion.

The 25-Day Healing Plan offers a structured, step-by-step approach to recovery, breaking down the process into manageable steps that focus on detoxification, gut repair, and long-term maintenance. Whether you're in the initial stages or in the final part of healing, consistency and patience are key.

Supplements, antibiotics, and probiotics are powerful tools that can help your recovery. By combining them with dietary changes and lifestyle modifications, you can rebuild a healthy gut microbiome and recover your digestive function.

Lifestyle factors such as stress control, sleep, and exercise play a pivotal role in the healing process. These practices support your immune system, improve gut motility, and lower inflammation, creating an optimal environment for healing.

Myths and misconceptions about SIBO can delay diagnosis and treatment. By addressing these misconceptions and knowing the facts, you are better prepared to navigate the complexities of this condition.

Working with healthcare providers is important. Collaboration, regular testing, and open communication ensure that your treatment plan stays effective and tailored to your unique needs.

Real-life success stories provide priceless insights into the recovery process. Hearing about the journeys of others who have successfully healed from SIBO offers both hope and practical tips for your own path to wellness.

Final Thoughts:

Healing from SIBO is not a one-size-fits-all method. It takes patience, commitment, and a willingness to listen to your body. While the road to recovery may have its ups and downs, the key is to remain consistent with your plan, change as needed, and maintain a positive, proactive attitude. Remember that you're not alone—countless people have successfully managed their SIBO, and with the right support and tools, you too can regain control of your gut health. It's important to accept the journey as a process of self-discovery and healing. By making informed choices, staying patient with your body's response, and continuing to educate yourself, you can experience lasting relief from SIBO and rebuild a healthy, vibrant life.

As you move forward, always remember: healing is possible, and your health is in your hands. Stay committed to the steps listed in this book, trust your healing process, and take things one day at a time. With the right attitude and tools, you will restore your gut health and live a life free from the constraints of SIBO.

Appendix

SIBO-Friendly Recipes

This section provides a collection of SIBO-friendly recipes designed to support your healing journey. All recipes follow the principles of the Low FODMAP or Specific Carbohydrate Diet (SCD), helping to reduce symptoms and promote gut health. These meals are nutritious, easy to prepare, and suitable for the various phases of your recovery plan.

1. SIBO-Friendly Chicken and Vegetable Soup
Ingredients:
- 1 chicken breast, diced
- 2 carrots, peeled and sliced
- 1 zucchini, sliced
- 1 cup spinach
- 2 cups chicken broth (low FODMAP)

- 1 tbsp olive oil

- Salt and pepper to taste

- Fresh herbs (optional)

Instructions:

1. In a large pot, heat olive oil and sauté diced chicken until browned.

2. Add the carrots, zucchini, and chicken broth. Bring to a boil.

3. Lower heat and simmer for 20 minutes, or until vegetables are tender.

4. Stir in the spinach and cook for an additional 5 minutes.

5. Season with salt, pepper, and fresh herbs. Serve warm.

2. Grilled Salmon with Lemon Herb Sauce

Ingredients:

- 1 salmon fillet

- 1 tbsp olive oil

- Juice of 1 lemon

- 1 garlic clove (optional, depending on tolerance)

- Fresh parsley, chopped

- Salt and pepper to taste

Instructions:

1. Preheat the grill or grill pan over medium heat.

2. Brush salmon with olive oil, lemon juice, and season with salt and pepper.

3. Grill the salmon for 4-6 minutes on each side or until it flakes easily with a fork.

4. While the salmon cooks, mix lemon juice, chopped parsley, and garlic in a small bowl (optional for SIBO sensitivity).

5. Drizzle the lemon herb sauce over the cooked salmon before serving.

3. SIBO-Friendly Roasted Sweet Potato with Avocado

Ingredients:

- 2 small sweet potatoes, peeled and cubed

- 1 avocado, sliced

- 1 tbsp olive oil

- Salt and pepper to taste

- Fresh cilantro (optional)

Instructions:

1. Preheat your oven to 400°F (200°C).

2. Toss cubed sweet potatoes with olive oil, salt, and pepper.

3. Roast the sweet potatoes on a baking sheet for 25-30 minutes or until soft and golden.

4. Once roasted, top with fresh avocado slices and cilantro.

5. Serve as a nutritious side dish or a light meal.

www.ingramcontent.com/pod-product-compliance
Lightning Source LLC
Chambersburg PA
CBHW051602250726
48653CB00004BA/1285